CHRONIC PAIN IN OLD AGE

An Integrated Biopsychosocial Perspective

Chronic pain is a daily fact of life for many elderly people. The pain is often seen as a product of age, and is only too readily accepted as inevitable by patient and physician.

This collection of original essays offers a comprehensive biopsychosocial approach to address the complex symptoms and treatment of chronic pain in the elderly. The nineteen contributors come from many disciplines, including psychology, medicine, social work, physical therapy, and nursing. Their primary objective is to improve the quality of pain management for seniors, but they also urge readers to examine their own attitudes and beliefs about elderly patients, to avoid the pitfalls of ageism and to refrain from using age to rationalize inaction.

The volume is loosely divided into three overlapping sections. The first addresses social, psychological, and epidemiological issues. The second section deals with family issues, including their role in pain management. The final section addresses psychological and medical interventions.

RANJAN ROY is a professor in the Faculty of Social Work and the Department of Psychiatry, University of Manitoba. He is author of numerous books, including *The Social Context of the Chronic Pain Sufferer*.

RANJAN ROY, EDITOR

Chronic Pain in Old Age: An Integrated Biopsychosocial Perspective

UNIVERSITY OF TORONTO PRESS
Toronto Buffalo London

© University of Toronto Press Incorporated 1995
Toronto Buffalo London
Printed in Canada
Reprinted in 2018
ISBN 0-8020-2859-4 (cloth)
ISBN 978-0-8020-7359-4 (paper)

∞

Printed on acid-free paper

Canadian Cataloguing in Publication Data

Main entry under title:

Chronic pain in old age : an integrated
biopsychosocial perspective

ISBN 0-8020-2859-4 (bound)   ISBN 978-0-8020-7359-4 (paper)

1. Pain in old age.   2. Chronic pain.
I. Roy, Ranjan.

RB127.C47 1995   616'.0472'084   C95-930171-2

University of Toronto Press acknowledges the financial assistance to its publishing
program of the Canada Council and the Ontario Arts Council.

To my parents, who passed through old age with grace

Contents

Section 3. Psychological and Medical Interventions

Foreword

Aches and pains are inevitable accompaniments of growing older. Most acute pains, such as periodic muscle or joint pains, are accepted as the consequences of maintaining an active, enjoyable life. Fortunately, they are also usually helped either by medications that are easily available or simply by relaxation and rest. Chronic pain, however, which is the special focus of this book, is the scourge of the elderly, just as it is for people of all ages. The particular tragedy for the elderly is the widespread belief that their pain is beyond help. The ageing process supposedly brings pain in its wake, and thre is nothing to do but suffer silently.

This book provides powerful arguments that this belief is simply not true: the elderly need not suffer pain any more than anyone else. In place of the passive, resigned attitude that the elderly are fated to suffer for merely surviving, health care providers are urged to take an active, dynamic approach to these pain problems. The varieties of pain in the elderly are not qualitatively unique; they are simply more common and sometimes more severe. With imagination and persistence, with positive attidues among the givers and receivers of pain management procedures, the elderly can be helped to a far greater extent than most of us have generally believed. This is as true for cancer pain as it is for arthritic pains, headaches, and the other aches and pains that plague people at every age, but reach a crescendo as we get older.

There has long been a need for a book on pain in the elderly that focuses on chronic pain and provides the information we need to cope with its special problems. Ranjan Roy presents us with an excellent book that covers virtually every major problem that faces the elderly and challenges professional caregivers. Section 1 deals with epidemiological, social, and psychological issues. Section 2 is concerned with family issues, which are so important in the attempt to deliver optimal care in a setting that provides the older person with the secuity of the family and familiar surroundings. Finally, Section 3 presents fascinating and useful evaluations of psychological and medical interventions.

The happy surprise to the reader of this book is how much knowledge we have already acquired in a field that has only recently begun to receive the attention it deserves. Professor Roy and the authors of these excellent chapters have made this information available to us in a well-organized volume. The book covers a broad field and does it interestingly and competently. Readers in all disciplines are certain to benefit. The valuable information in this book should lead to less suffering in the elderly. Here is another opportunity to combat the tragedy of needless pain.

This book reveals Professor Roy's skills as an editor. He has highlighted an important problem that needs urgently to be addressed, chosen knowledgeable and competent contributors, and provided a vehicle for informative, valuable chapters. This book is an important contribution to knowledge in the growing field of pain in the elderly and is certain to provide a powerful impetus to its continuing growth and importance.

Ronald Melzack
E.P. Taylor Professor
McGill University
Montreal, Canada

Preface

Inevitable as old age is, to be old in our society is not without problems and prejudices. Some years ago a young colleague made a presentation of his successfully defended PhD thesis. His central finding was that post-retirement adjustment for a group of retirees in their late sixties in a small English town was excellent. This young scholar was almost ridiculed for his 'bizarre' finding. Serious methodological inadequacies in his study were discussed. The central objection of this learned audience was that happiness and contentment were incongruent with old age and retirement. The truth of the matter was that contentment and advancing years were widely accepted as incompatible. Now, we are more willing to agree, based on empirical evidence, that retirement is much less of a crisis for many. Indeed, often early retirement is eagerly sought. Others are happy to retire from hard labouring and often unpleasant jobs and still others from jobs that are inherently stressful. Erich Fromm in his essay 'The Psychological Problems of Aging' wrote, 'The older person, let us say after sixty-five, really has a chance to live, to be alive, to make a living his main business. He can also confront himself genuinely with the spiritual and religious problems of life. I think that in the past history of humanity men usually had no energy or no time left to be seriously concerned with such problems.' Old age and the pursuit of knowledge and happiness need not be incompatible.

Pain, unfortunately, is a daily fact of life for many elderly persons. Arthritic diseases account for much of that pain. Perhaps because of the pervasiveness of pain in this population, pain is not always well managed. With increasing age the brain's capacity to feel pain goes down – or, so it is said. Pain in old age is often taken for granted. In my work I see elderly patients who are fatalistic about their pain. In almost every chapter of this volume concern is expressed about many misconceptions that continue to flourish in the treatment and management of pain in the elderly. If indeed there is a common theme that provides continuity to this book, it is the collective plea of every contributor that we examine our attitudes and beliefs about our elderly patients, avoid the pitfall of ageism, and refrain from finding explanation for our inaction in the age of our patients.

Pain in the elderly has also been subjected to much stereotyping. Our own research has shown that elderly patients themselves show a certain amount of resignation in their acceptance of, at times, even severe pain. To be old is to silently tolerate pain. Health care professionals also feed into this myth. The myth has two faces. One, that old age and pain are predestined to coexist and second, because of this predestination, not much can be done to control or ameliorate this pain. Both, of course, are untrue. More variability in the health status is to be found in the elderly population than in any other age group. Most people do not survive to see their eightieth birthday. Yet, those who do, and the number is substantial and on the rise, may and do enjoy good health and good cheer.

The idea for this book evolved over several years. Our own research on pain in the elderly, our clinical observations, and greater attention to this topic in the recent literature all contributed to the ultimate shape of this volume. My initial plan was to focus exclusively on psychological and social issues of pain in the elderly for the simple reason that these two areas are quite neglected in the clinical literature. I abandoned that line of thinking to avoid one of the major gaps in the pain literature on the elderly – the absence of a comprehensive biopsychosocial approach to address the complex presentation and treatment of chronic pain in the elderly.

The perspective of this book is inter- and multidisciplinary. This is reflected both in the wide range of academic disciplines of the contributors and in the topics themselves. Psychology, medicine, social work, physical therapy, and nursing are represented in this volume. Occupational therapy is the obvious omission, but that is not entirely due to lack of trying. In fact, finding contributors for this book became a major undertaking. I consulted widely with my friends and colleagues in Canada, the United States, the United Kingdom, Australia, New Zealand, France, and Sweden. The common response was that very few 'experts' were to be found in the field of pain in the elderly. Despite that shortcoming, an impressive group of experts were located who agreed to participate in this project. The contributors to this volume are concerned clinicians and researchers whose primary objective is to improve the quality of pain management for the elderly.

This volume is divided into three, somewhat overlapping, sections. The first section has four chapters, and, in broad terms, they address social, psychological, and epidemiological issues. Prevalence and some management issues are discussed in the foundation chapter by Margaret Ross and Joan Crook. Epidemiological studies are few, but these authors, by drawing on a very broad literature, convey a clear sense of the magnitude of the problem. They also provide an excellent summary of some of the social, psychological, and medical aspects of pain management in the elderly.

In chapter 2, Andrew Cook and I undertake the daunting task of exploring the attitudes and beliefs about pain in the elderly. We draw on our own clinical experience, our research, and the limited literature that exists on the subject to make this somewhat unwieldy area clinically relevant. The central point is that no single attitude or belief is shared by all elderly individuals about the cause of their pain nor, for that matter, is there a single attitude towards finding a solution. Without question, old age has an influence in shaping attitudes and beliefs about pain and illness. The point to remember is that these attitudes and beliefs are quite varied.

Pain is an extraordinarily common symptom in the elderly. Michael Thomas, my friend and associate, mainly drawing on our own research on pain in healthy elderly, addresses the key issues about pain perception, attitudes, and help-seeking behaviour in the elderly, who frequently live with and tolerate very painful conditions. This population does not frequent medical clinics and is, in the main, quite unaware of the existence of pain clinics in their community. Bruce Sorkin and Dennis Turk provide a logical follow-up on the previous chapter by focusing on the pain issues in the young vis-à-vis the elderly. They are very persuasive in making a case for the adoption of psychological approaches to manage pain in the elderly. A multitude of reasons are offered to deny the elderly the benefits of cognitive pain management. Sorkin and Turk, based on their research and clinical experience, successfully refute the ageism that often results in poor treatment of pain in the elderly.

Section 2 has two chapters dealing with family issues. In Chapter 5, I review the broad literature on family therapy with the elderly medically ill patients. Specific literature on family issues dealing with the elderly pain sufferer is almost non-existent. A case of a man with herpes zoster is presented to show the benefits that might accrue from short-term couple therapy. Betty Ferrell and Lynne Rivera in Chapter 6 discuss the role of the family in the management of pain in cancer patients. This is the only chapter in this volume that deals with cancer pain. Ferrell's research is ground breaking and has much to teach us about how family members can be successfully engaged in the endeavour to improve the quality of life not only for the patients, but also for those who take care of them.

The third and final section, dealing with psychological and medical interventions, has five chapters. Psychological and medical interventions, though examined separately in individual chapters, constitute an integral part of treatment, and a body–mind division is recognised by all as undesirable.

In Chapter 7 Steve Harkins and his colleagues explain not only some of the current thinking on pain mechanisms, but also the psychoneurological factors that complicate the clinical presentation of pain in the elderly. Furthermore, they provide clinical guidelines to assess pain in this population and make a strong case for a comprehensive approach to pain management. In Chapter 8 Steve Aung brings to bear the fruits of his extensive knowledge of Chinese medicine. He reviews the role of pain clinics in the management and treatment of pain in elderly patients. By combining the ancient knowledge of Chinese medicine with modern Western medicine, Aung demonstrates the value of his approach in successfully treating a variety of painful conditions that afflict his elderly patients. Guy Vendendries, in Chapter 9, gives us the benefit of his vast experience of running an in-patient geriatric program. Management of pain is a key focus of his program. Vendendries provides a detailed account of what may constitute the 'dos' and 'don'ts' of pain management in the geriatric population. Vendendries wrote his chapter in French, and I take full responsibility for the translated version – recognizing that in the process of translation some of the subtleties and nuances may have been lost; I would like to believe, however, that the chapter is a very close approximation of the original.

Chapters 10 and 11 are concerned with psychiatric and psychological problems and their management. Pam Melding delineates some of the major as well as the lesser psychiatric illnesses in the geriatric population and examines their relationship with the experience of pain. The relationships between medical illnesses and their psychiatric manifestations and vice versa are explored. Melding's careful analyses of somatoform disorders in the elderly is especially useful, as these problems tend to be minimized in the elderly population. She urges careful evaluation of psychiatric problems in the context of pain and their proper management in this somewhat overlooked population. Finally, in Chapter 11, Don Bakal and his colleagues share their unique experience of helping their patients cope more effectively with pain through 'somatic awareness.' They provide several case illustrations to show the effectiveness of their approach with elderly patients.

This volume is the product of the very hard work of dedicated clinicians

and researchers. To a person, they are an extremely busy group of individuals. That I was successful in persuading them to take out a great deal of
time to write leaves me in their debt. Professor Ronald Melzack very kindly
agreed to write the Foreword, for which he has my gratitude.

Ranjan Roy
Winnipeg, Manitoba
January 1994

Contributors

Foreword: Professor Ronald Melzack, FRSC, Department of Psychology, McGill University, Montreal, Canada.

Stephen K.H. Aung, MD, Clinical Assistant Professor, Department of Family Medicine, University of Alberta, Edmonton, Alberta, Canada.

Donald Bakal, PhD, Professor, Department of Psychology, University of Calgary, Calgary, Alberta, Canada.

Andrew Cook, MA, Doctoral Student, Department of Psychology, University of Manitoba, Winnipeg, Manitoba, Canada.

Joan M. Crook, RN, PhD, Professor, School of Nursing, Faculty of Health Sciences, McMaster University, Hamilton, Ontario, Canada.

Betty Ferrell, PhD, City of Hope Hospital, Duarte, California, USA.

Stephen W. Harkins, PhD, Professor, Department of Gerontology, Medical College of Virginia, Virginia Commonwealth University, Richmond, Virginia, USA.

Belinda T. Lagua, BS, P.T. Holbein Place, Richmond, Virginia, USA.

Peter Meiring, MD, Southern Alberta Regional Geriatric Center, Calgary, Canada.

Pamela Melding, MD, North Shore Hospital, Private Bag Takapuna, New Zealand.

D.D. Price, PhD, Department of Anesthesiology, Virginia Commonwealth University, Richmond, Virginia, USA.

Lynne M. Rivera, BSc, RN, City of Hope Hospital, Duarte, California, USA.

Margaret M. Ross, RN, PhD, School of Nursing, University of Ottawa, Ottawa, Ontario, Canada.

Ranjan Roy, Professor, Faculty of Social Work and Department of Psychiatry, University of Manitoba, Winnipeg, and Consultant

(Scientific), Department of Anesthesia, St Boniface Hospital, Winnipeg, Canada.

Ralph E. Small, PharmD, Department of Pharmacy, Virginia Commonwealth University, Richmond, Virginia, USA.

Bruce A. Sorkin, PhD, Pain Evaluation and Treatment Institute, Pittsburgh, Pennsylvania, USA.

Elaine Stokes, MD, Southern Alberta Regional Geriatric Center, Calgary, Canada.

Michael Thomas, PhD, Associate Professor, Department of Psychology, University of Manitoba, Winnipeg, Canada.

Dennis C. Turk, PhD, Professor, Department of Psychiatry, University of Pittsburgh and Director, Pain Evaluation and Treatment Institute, Pittsburgh, Pennsylvania, USA.

Guy Vandendries, MD, Clinique Médicale de la Porte Verte, Versailles, France.

Section 1

Social, Psychological, and Epidemiological Issues

1

Pain in Later Life:
Present State of Knowledge

MARGARET M. ROSS and JOAN M. CROOK

The purpose of this chapter is to increase awareness, through a review of the existing research, of the importance of pain in later life and to explore what is known of its prevalence and its relationship to disability and independent living. As Canada enters the twenty-first century, the population aged sixty-five and over will escalate to nearly four million people. It will further escalate to six million or 20 per cent of the population by 2021 and by another 1.5 million to one-quarter (23.8 per cent) of the population by the year 2031 (Statistics Canada, 1990). Older adults are at a point in their lives where the onset of illness of a life-threatening nature and/or chronic illness and disability are expected. Ageing is also accompanied by social and psychological changes, many of which are thought to contribute to the way that older adults experience pain.

Although the association between pain and disability in later life is unclear, pain is known to be a factor that propels individuals to seek medical attention (Crook, Rideout, and Browne, 1984). Given the rising costs of health care, efforts to prevent disabling pain and to facilitate the development of independent living in later life are crucial. Nevertheless, pain as an aspect of illness or other changes in later life is a relatively neglected area of research. Knowledge regarding its prevalence is scarce and contradictory, and little is known about its relationship to disability and independent living.

A NEGLECTED AREA OF RESEARCH

The reasons for the dearth of epidemiological research related to pain in the elderly are many. Older adults are, in large measure, excluded from paid labour (work forces many in pain to seek help), and many live in poverty (rendering them ineligible for many types of pain therapy). The myths and stereotypes associated with ageing, held not only by older adults themselves but also by health care workers, support the belief that pain in later life is predestined and unavoidable. Older adults who internalize the view that pain is a normal component of ageing may fail to report or under-report their pain. They may also expect that professionals *know* how much pain they are experiencing or are fearful of the meaning of their pain and the outcomes of treatment. In addition, the misguided notions that age dulls the ability to perceive pain or that elderly people complain more about pain than their younger counterparts do underscore the reported tendency of many health care workers to deny or minimize the pain experience of elderly patients. Nurses, for example, have been reported to assess less pain in older burn patients when compared with those who are young (Van Der Does, 1989). There are also reports that older adults receive less analgesic medication following surgery or for cancer pain than do their younger counterparts (Thienhaus, 1989). With good reason, the literature is replete with warnings about the susceptibility of older adults to medications, their side-effects, and their interactions. Nevertheless, fears of over-medication, the possibility of addiction, and a lack of knowledge on the part of prescribers and dispensers of medications often results in inadequate pain control among older adults. Contrary to erroneous beliefs that narcotic medications are inappropriate for patients with non-malignant pain and that the potential side-effects of narcotic analgesics preclude their use with elderly individuals, these medications may be used safely with older adults.

Research into pain and ageing is also inhibited by the small proportion of older patients who are admitted to pain clinics (Harkins, 1988) and consequently available as research subjects. For these reasons and others, little is known of the prevalence of pain and its effects on older adults.

PRESENT STATE OF KNOWLEDGE

Pain and ageing studies focus on seniors living either in the community or in institutions. Much of what is known of pain in later life derives from the work of researchers who did not set out to study elderly persons specifically, but included in their samples a substantial proportion of respondents who were over the age of sixty-five. In general, an overview of the literature on pain and ageing provides evidence that when asked about pain, between 73 and 80 per cent of older respondents admit to its presence (Demlow, Liang, and Eaton, 1986; Thomas and Roy, 1988).

Older adults dwelling in the community. One epidemiological study that provided information about the prevalence of pain among older adults involved a random survey of 500 households in Burlington, Ontario (Crook et al., 1984). Findings from this study revealed that age-specific morbidity rates for persistent pain increased with age. Persistent pain was defined as pain which was 'often or usually present and having occurred within the last two weeks.' Morbidity associated with pain among those over the age of sixty-five was twice (250 per thousand) that found in younger respondents (125 per thousand). Age-specific rates for persistent pain were 19.9 per cent in the sixth decade of life, 25 per cent in the seventh, 29 per cent in the eighth decade, and 40 per cent in those over the age of eighty.

Another large study (Harris et al., 1985) surveyed 1,254 adults, including 200 who were sixty-five and over. By contrast, this study found younger people to report more pain, specifically pain associated with headache, backache, muscle pain, stomach pain, and dental pain. In this study, only joint pain was more frequent for older persons. In a study by Roy and Thomas (1986) of a random sample of 205 elderly subjects, who were by all accounts relatively healthy and belonged to a network of social clubs, nearly 70 per cent reported having some kind of pain problem. Sorkin, Rudy, Hanlon, Turk, and Stieg (1990) compared younger (age thirty-five or younger) and older (age sixty-five or older) patients referred to a chronic pain clinic and observed no differences between the two groups in pain severity ratings. These studies highlight the need for clarification of the issue of pain in later life.

Older adults in institutions. Studies of pain among nursing home residents suggest that over 70 per cent of this frail elderly population have significant pain problems. Roy and Thomas (1986) surveyed ninety-seven nursing home residents ranging in age from sixty-five to eighty and found that 83 per cent reported current pain problems. Fifty per cent of subjects reported low levels of pain, 21 per cent moderate levels, and 18 per cent high to intolerable levels. The majority of respondents in this study reported pain of at least two years' duration. Ferrell, Ferrell, and Osterwell (1990) reported that 71 per cent of ninety-seven residents of a multilevel nursing home had pain. Their study documented the significant relationships among pain, functional status, and overall quality of life. Some of the adverse effects of pain reported by respondents were: impaired enjoyable activities (recreational and social events), impaired ambulation (walking, transfers), impaired posture, sleep disturbances, depressed affect, and functional disturbances such as constipation and incontinence. These studies suggest that there may be a tendency to underestimate the prevalence and intensity of pain in older residents of nursing homes.

A Canadian study of 2,415 randomly selected subjects described the prevalence, consequence, and resolution of pain in hospitalized patients (Abott et al., 1992). The researchers reported that pain of longer duration was significantly associated with increasing age and female gender. As a result of pain, patients reported difficulty moving (50 to 66 per cent), sleeping (38 to 50 per cent), eating (22 to 33 per cent), concentrating (34 to 54 per cent), and talking (25 to 36 per cent), as well as nervousness (44 to 53 per cent) and distress (37 to 45 per cent) over the interviews during hospitalization, and follow-up at three weeks, three months, and six months.

The Last Year of Life

The study of pain during the last phase of life and as an aspect of the dying process of older adults, while fraught with methodological and ethical difficulties, has been undertaken. A retrospective study by Cartwright, Hockey, and Anderson (1973) investigated the last year of life of a random sample of 785 persons aged fifteen and over, the majority (70 per cent) of whom were over the age of sixty-five. While these researchers found a tendency for pain to be somewhat less for the older age group, of those over the age of sixty-five, close to two-thirds (64 per cent) were reported to have pain in their final year.

A hospice study of cancer patients, the majority (two-thirds) of whom were over the age of sixty-five, found that 17 per cent of kin informants reported pain at the most severe level at six weeks prior to the patient's death (Mor, 1987; Morris, Mor, Goldberg, Sherwood, Greer, and Hiris, 1986a; Morris, Suissa, Sherwood, Wright, and Greer, 1986b). This compared with 25 per cent within two days of death.

A more recent study by Moss and Lawton of 200 deceased older community-dwelling residents found that pain increased over the final year of life. Data were gathered retrospectively from the nearest relative six months after the subject's death. These researchers reported that 37 per cent of subjects were described as having had pain in the last twelve months of their lives and that one month before death 66 per cent felt pain frequently or all the time.

In a summary of existing research, Melding (1992) concluded that epidemiological studies of pain in later life are limited and that their findings can be summarized as follows: (a) the incidence of chronic pain does increase with advancing age; (b) chronic pain is a common problem, and most studies suggest a prevalence of about 30 to 40 per cent in older adults, and this rises in the terminal phase of life; (c) much chronic pain is associated with physical illness, and this is also more common in old age; (d) most of the available studies have surveyed the younger old (sixty-five to seventy-five), who perceive pain similarly to younger adults, but data on the old (seventy-five plus) are seriously deficient; and (e) there are suggestions that the perception of pain may decrease in extreme old age or near death.

PAIN, DISABILITY, AND AGEING

The importance of pain and ageing as an area of research derives, in part, from its association with disability and quality of life. The literature on ageing and disability focuses primarily on mortality and morbidity. The study of mortality provides information about problems that threaten life; the study of morbidity provides information about problems that affect quality of life.

Mortality. The three most significant causes of death in the elderly population are cardiovascular disease, cancer, and respiratory disease for men and heart disease, cancer, and cerebrovascular disease for women (Statistics Canada, 1990). There is anecdotal, clinical, and emerging research evidence that these diseases are associated with varying degrees of pain. For example, with respect to cardiovascular disease, until recently, it was thought that age was associated with a decrease in pain. More recent evidence, however, suggests otherwise. In a study of 1,474 patients admitted to a coronary care unit, it was demonstrated that pain was the most frequent presenting symptom in the majority of patients being treated for myocardial infarction (MacDonald, Baillie, Willian, and Ballantyne, 1983). According to another researcher (Harkins, 1988), angina and precordial pain show increasing frequency with increasing age. Foley (1985) has demonstrated that cancer is an important source of pain among older people. In fact, according to Witte (1989), the primary source of information on pain in later life derives from the cancer literature. With respect to cerebrovascular disease, Melding (1991) has noted that severe intractable pain frequently accompanies stroke, as infarction destroys sensory pathways.

Morbidity. The prevalence of chronic health problems among elderly persons lends further credence to the notion that pain is a problem that many must cope with in their later years. Brody and Kleban (1983), using a log format, investigated the physical and mental health symptoms of 120 older people and noted that 73 per cent reported pain of some kind. It is estimated that 80 per cent of those over the age of sixty-five suffer from at least one chronic illness (Harkins, Kwentus, and Price, 1984; Osburn, Simmons Tropea, and Schwenger, 1986; Kane, Ouslander, and Ouslander, 1989). Many of these are physical in nature (arthritis, osteoporosis, peripheral vascular disease, polymyalgia rheumatica, intermittent claudication, herpes zoster or shingles, and others) and are associated with pain, discomfort, and suffering. Other chronic illnesses are mental and/or cognitive in nature and may also be associated with pain and suffering, or they may mask the symptoms of pain. The symptom of pain, regardless of its etiology, is also associated with sleep disturbance, fatigue, emotional distress, and functional and social disability. These co-morbid factors add to the burden of illness.

Physical Disorders. There are a plethora of physical disorders with which older people may be afflicted, including musculoskeletal and joint disorders, headache, abdominal complaints, and cancer.

Musculoskeletal and joint conditions that cause pain occur frequently among older adults (Kane and Ouslander, 1989). Valkenburg (1988) found that 30 per cent of men and 53 per cent of women over the age of fifty-five experienced peripheral joint pain. Indeed, Harris et al. (1985) reported that only pain associated with joints increases with age, a finding that Melding (1992: 2) labels as 'surprising since up to 80% of older adults have one chronic health problem that may be associated with pain.' Most amputations also occur in this age group (Butler, 1991). Stelian, Gil, Habot, Rosenthal, Abramovici, Kutok, and Khakit (1992) reported that back pain resulting from osteoarthritis is a frequent occurrence among older adults. Twenty-four per cent of women and 18.4 per cent of men with arthritic changes report back pain. Based on respondents' self-reports, Von Korff (1988) estimated that among persons surviving to age seventy, 85 per cent will experience a problem of back pain. In addition, there are reports of shoulder pain (Warren and O'Brien, 1989), low back pain (Vanharanta, Sachs, Ohnmeiss, and, April, 1989), and neurological pain (Tunks, 1988) in the elderly population. Hip fractures peak in the eighth decade of life (Brummel-Smith, 1990). Harkins (1988) speculated that it was likely that considerable long-term morbidity and perhaps mortality in later life re-sulted from the stress of pain accompanying fractures.

Headaches are another cause of pain, the prevalence of which varies dramatically with age, according to Lipton, Pfeffer, Newman, and Solomon, 1993. These authors report that while primary headache disorders, such as migraine and cluster, decline with age, secondary headache disorders, in-cluding temporal arteritis and mass lesions, increase. A prevalence rate for migraine headaches of 5 per cent in women and 10 per cent in men age seventy and over compared with 30 and 10 per cent respectively in younger counterparts has been reported in one population survey (Stewart, Lipton, Celentano, and Reed, 1992). It is furthermore reported that tension-type headaches increased with age with a prevalence of 27 per cent in persons over the age of sixty-five (Solomon, Kunkel, and Frame, 1990). There is also at least one primary headache disorder unique to older people, the hypnic headache syndrome (Raskin, 1988; Newman, Lipton, and Soloman, 1991). The age of onset for this headache syndrome ranges from sixty-five to eighty-four, and patients present with headaches that awaken them at the same time every night for fifteen to sixty minutes. Because the use of medication increases with age, drugs are also an important secondary cause of headaches in older adults.

Abdominal disorders may be an important cause of pain in later life. Bugliosi, Meloy, and Vukov (1990) conducted a one-year retrospective study of 127 elderly patients ranging in age from sixty-eight to ninety-one who presented to an emergency department with acute non-traumatic abdominal pain. The most common diagnosis arrived at in the emergency room was indeterminate abdominal pain (24 per cent). Biliary tract disease (12 per cent) and small bowel obstruction (12 per cent) were the most common specific diagnoses. Of the fifty-four patients (42.5 per cent) who were admitted for observation or medical management, twenty-two (41 per cent) eventually required surgical intervention. All in all, 17.3 per cent of the 127 patients studied required surgery for their abdominal pain. The researchers made a plea for liberal admission policies for older adults presenting at an emergency department with abdominal pain.

Cancer is a much feared disorder known to emerge in later life. Indeed, much of the work on pain and ageing derives from studies of cancer and the hospice movement. A descriptive and exploratory study of home hospice patients by Dobratz, Burns, and Oden (1987) and a study of pain management in a home hospice program by Byrd, Taylor, and Altmiller (1987) provided information about the pain experience of older adults with cancer. The mean age of respondents for both studies was over sixty-five, and results demonstrated that pain was a problem for a substantial proportion of patients, as was the resolution of their pain. The limitation of these data to cancer patients in a hospice setting clearly prevents any generalization regarding pain prevalence or its change as death nears. Nevertheless, these findings concur with other studies that suggest that 25 per cent of patients with cancer throughout the world suffer from severe pain at the time of death (Twycross and Lack, 1983) and that 20 to 100 per cent of patients experience considerable pain during the time before death (Greenwald, Bonica, and Bergner, 1987).

In summary, physical disorders are but one mechanism that can assist in the explanation of pain in later life. Ageing is also accompanied by changes of a social and psychological nature, many of which are thought to contribute to the perception and perpetuation of pain (Melding, 1991). Among these are depression and cognitive impairment.

Pain and Depression

Although the interaction of pain and emotion has been a controversial issue for many years (Turk and Rudy, 1986), there is research evidence of an association between chronic pain and psychological distress, particularly depression (see Chapter 10). A number of studies have shown that chronic pain patients report greater depression than do other individuals (Romano and Turner, 1985; Roy, Thomas, and Matas, 1984). Magni, Schtano, and Deleo, 1985) investigated complaints of joint pain and found a significant association with depression. Parmelee, Katz, and Lawton (1991) investigated 568 institutionalized elderly people and found that those who had major depressive illness (DSM-IIIR criteria) reported more intense pain than did those who were not depressed. Pain was even more likely to be endorsed in these patients if there was a physical disorder relevant to the particular pain problem. Mansfield and Marx (1993) investigated the relationship between depressed affect and pain in a secondary analysis of data on 408 nursing home residents. Cognitive impairment, activities of daily living impairment, quality of social networks, and a number of medical diagnoses were also assessed. Analysis revealed that depressed residents were more likely to have pain, regardless of the presence of cognitive impairment. According to Melding (1992; see Chapter 10), overall, most studies that have explored chronic pain patients have found an incidence of depressive illness in 30 to 50 per cent of them. This effect is correlated with the illness and degree of pain and is independent of age.

Many explanations have been offered for the relationship between pain and depression. Romano and Turner (1985) concluded that there was research support for virtually all (often contradictory) hypotheses about the nature of the pain and depression relationship. Tunks (1990) reviewed the evidence regarding the relationship of pain and psychological disorders and concluded that there was no one stereotypical chronic pain syndrome, but rather many chronic pain problems that because of various factors take various forms. It seems reasonable, however, to hypothesize that activity restriction associated with declining mobility and increasing dependence in later life may account for a significant portion of the association between pain and depression among older adults. Pain may influence depressed affect primarily in the extent that it results in activity restriction and functional limitations (Gamsa, 1990). Underlying this reasoning is the assumption that pain is an important contributor to functional disability and that difficulty in conducting routine activities, recreation, and family and work role functions would contribute to depressed affect. There is also suggestive evidence of this relationship in a study of elderly out-patients who reside in the community (Williamson and Schultz, 1992).

Pain and Cognitive Impairment

Although several sensory systems do decline in later life, and the incidence of moderate to severe dementia is approximately 5 to 7 per cent for those between the ages of sixty-five and eighty and 20 per cent thereafter (Melding, 1992), little is known of whether organic brain impairment influences the pain threshold and if it does – how? The perception and communication of pain is in part dependent on the cognitive–evaluative component of brain function. Older adults who have problems with attention, memory, and concentration ability may be unable to localize, discriminate, and/or describe their pain. The resulting distress of unexpressed and unresolved pain has the potential of resulting in confusion and aggressive behaviour. Complicating the issue of pain assessment in those who are confused and non-verbal is the fact that most pain assessment tools rely on verbal reports of pain. Indeed, little attention has been devoted to determining if tools used to measure pain are valid and reliable with elderly populations (Herr and Mobility, 1993). According to Melding (1992), on the one hand, pain is frequently a complaint in early dementia, and there is a tendency to erroneously perceive sensory stimuli that may be somatized. On the other hand, pain complaints may obscure cognitive impairment (Anderson, Kaplan, and Falsenthal 1992). Illness is only one mechanism through which complaints of pain in old age can be understood. There are suggestions in the literature that personal history, birth cohort, and psychological disposition are factors that influence both the experience and the reporting of pain (Harkins, 1988).

Because the majority of elderly individuals experience at least one chronic illness, care must be taken to avoid attributing acute pain to pre-existing chronic illnesses (see Chapter 10). Many older adults may not report pain because they do not want to bother anyone. Additionally, the meaning of pain is known to be influenced by life experience, including role transitions, pain memories, and personal style (Melding, 1992). Knowledge of pain and ageing is rudimentary and fraught with unanswered questions. The problematic nature of current research renders this area of research potentially fruitful for gerontologists, pain researchers, and those interested in the quality of life of older adults.

PROBLEMATIC NATURE OF CURRENT RESEARCH

Studies have shown that pain impairment in later life is a common and costly problem, but accurate and precise estimates of the burden of illness and disability are difficult to make. Discrepancies in the prevalence of figures among studies are largely the result of differences in the classification of a 'case,' the measurement of the severity, frequency, and duration of pain, sampling frameworks, and survey techniques.

The heterogeneity of the older population must be reflected in research initiatives aimed at providing information about the prevalence and experience of pain among older adults, who differ more from one another than do the members of any other age group. For the most part, however, research on pain and ageing focuses on the experience of those who are institutionalized or living independently in their homes. The prevalence and severity of pain among those who are maintaining their independence at home with the assistance of visiting nurses and other home support services is not apparent in the literature. In addition, the prevalence of pain among those who are very old, nanely, over the age of eighty-five, is unknown. Additionally, the extent to which pain is related to physical, social, and emotional function, and the resources and strategies that older persons use to manage their pain are unknown.

Other problematic aspects relate to the contradictory and somewhat confusing nature of research results, even regarding the pain threshold in later life. On the one hand, there are suggestions that pain thresholds increase with age. One study found that 35 per cent of patients over the age of sixty with demonstrable gastric ulcers had no symptoms (Clinch, Banerjee, and Ostick, 1984). Another study reported that older adults were also less likely to complain of chest pain when experiencing acute heart attacks (Bayer, Joginder, Raafat, and Pathy, 1986). Whether these findings represent a change in threshold, physiology, psychology, reporting, or tolerance is unknown. On the other hand, studies suggest that both threshold and tolerance decrease with age, and that the aged become less able to perceive, differentiate, and accurately report pain (Sheridan, 1992).

Some other findings provide confusing direction for the practice of health care providers. For example, the Nuprin survey (Harris et al., 1985) suggested that only pain associated with joints increased with age. Melding (1991) expressed surprise at this result, because up to 80 per cent of older adults have at least one chronic health problem that may be associated with pain. In contrast, Harkins (1988) reviewed data collected from 86,000 patients, many of whom were over the age of sixty-five, who visited five family practice centres. He concluded that pain problems associated with musculoskeletal and cardiovascular systems increased with advancing age. This survey also found that the spectrum of painful conditions changed in old age. While headaches and some forms of back pain became less frequent, pain associated with osteoarthritis, rheumatism, angina, and vascular disease became more prevalent. These findings concur with those of Crook et al. (1984) who found that morbidity for pain increases with age.

THE ASSESSMENT AND MANAGEMENT OF PAIN IN LATER LIFE

It has been said that pain is most poorly managed in those who are most defenceless against it – the young and the elderly (Liebeskind and Melzack, 1987). Given the present state of knowledge regarding pain in later life, it is not surprising that the literature is primarily descriptive and anecdotal in nature. In assessing and managing pain in older adults, it is crucial that complaints of pain not be viewed and treated as a normal process of ageing.

Assessment. Pain is whatever the person says it is, and all complaints of pain should result in a careful diagnostic assessment, including a review of the individual's medication history. Tunks (1988) suggests that since multiple drugs may cloud the medical portrait of older adults, a period of detoxification may be necessary. Information about the onset, duration, quality, intensity, as well as the precipitating, exacerbating, and relieving factors, needs to be gathered. However, this is not always as easy as it sounds.

Herr and Mobility (1993) described the complexities of gathering and interpreting information about pain in older adults, including sensory deficits, difficulty with language, and myths and stereotypes held by older persons themselves, and they provided suggestions for adaptations to facilitate accurate and reliable assessment. Although a variety of tools are available for gathering data about specific aspects of pain, few of these tools have been validated with an elderly population. Herr and Mobility (1993) suggest that the Visual Analogue Scale may be too abstract for elderly persons in acute pain, with lower educational levels, impaired cognition, or impaired motor coordination. These authors also suggest that the McGill Pain Questionnaire, because of its length, complexity, and time-consuming characteristics, may be difficult for older adults to understand and tolerate. The MPQ body chart, however, seems to be an effective way of determining the location and quality of pain in those who have difficulty verbally describing their pain. They also refer to tools adapted from those used with children for elderly persons who are non-verbal. The use of a daily diary is advocated by Haley and Dafoe (1986) to identify activities or stressors linked to pain. It is crucial that appropriate methods of assessment be developed that are sensitive to the specific characteristics of the elderly population. The accurate assessment of pain is critical for the identification of appropriate intervention and for the evaluation of strategies aimed at controlling pain in those who are elderly.

Intervention. The management of pain involves both psychosocial and pharmacological interventions. Those of a psychosocial nature, however, are not used as frequently as they should be, because younger professionals may view problems of older adults as overly complex and demanding (Tunks, 1988). Behavioural techniques such as biofeedback, operant reinforcement strategies and cognitive behavioural strategies, can make a significant contribution to the relief of pain in older adults.

Although pharmacological treatment is a basic component of pain control, physiological changes associated with ageing must be considered when prescribing drugs. Older adults are more sensitive to the pain-relieving effects of narcotics and are more likely to suffer side-effects at lower doses than are younger people. The safety margin between therapeutic and toxic levels is also narrower in the elderly (Kwentus, Harkins, Lignon, and Silverman, 1985).

Sloan (1992) provides a list of guidelines that should underlie prescribing practices for older adults. These include minimizing or simplifying medication regimes, determining the efficacy of the medications prescribed, observing for adverse drug reactions, and assuming responsibility for knowing the changes associated with ageing and their potential impact on prescribing practices. Additionally, he suggests that patient functioning is indispensable as an end-point and that drug treatment that does not increase independence is probably not worth the risk of drug interactions, adverse effects, and compliance problems. While not advocating the overzealous discontinuation of helpful medication, the author advocates using the smallest number of medications that will achieve a satisfactory level of activities of daily living. Older adults should not be denied adequate analgesia for fear of side-effects, but rather should be monitored closely for their development.

CONCLUSION

The health and well-being of older adults is predicated on living in relative comfort and independence. Pain as an aspect of later life is a phenomenon about which much remains to be learned. The rising costs of health care, particularly with an ageing population, are of national concern. Seniors, particularly those over the age of seventy-five, are among the highest consumers of health care services. They are frequently in receipt of multiple medications and other treatments that may be redundant or conflicting and result in iatrogenic complications.

The hospitalization rates for older adults are markedly higher than for younger age groups. Consultations with physicians and nurses are also known to increase with age. Per capita health care expenditures for seniors average four times those of other age groups. Although a variety of predisposing factors (e.g., age, gender, beliefs, attitudes, ethnicity), enabling issues (e.g., lack of spouse or children, rural residence, availability of health care workers), and need factors (e.g., subjective perceptions and objective diagnosis) influence the rate of health care utilization, most studies indicate that need factors are the most important in determining whether hospital services or physicians will be used by older adults (Chappell, Strain, and Blanford, 1986). It seems reasonable to suggest that the decreased functioning associated with advancing age may be a result not only of disability, but also of pain. It would also appear beneficial to individuals and society in general to be able to accurately determine and successfully manage pain in later life.

REFERENCES

Abbott, F.V., Gray-Donald, K., Sewitch, M.J. Johnston, C.C., Edgar L., & Jeans, M.E. (1992). The prevalence of pain in hospitalized patients and resolution over six months. *Pain, 50*, 15–28.

Anderson, J.M., Kaplan, M.S., & Falsenthal, G. (1992). Brain injury obscured by chronic pain: A preliminary report. *Archives of Physical and Medical Rehabilitation, 71*, 703–8.

Bayer, A.J., Joginder, S.C., Raafat, R.F., & Pathy, S.J. (1986). Changing presentations of myocardial infarctions with increasing old age. *Journal of the American Geriatric Society, 34,* 263–6.

Brody, E., & Kleban, M. (1983). Day to day: Mental and physical health symptoms of older people: A report on health logs. *Gerontologist, 23,* 75–85.

Brummel-Smith, K. (1990). Rehabilitation. In: C.K. Cassel, D.E. Riesenberg, L.B. Sorenson, & J.R.Walsh (Eds.), *Geriatric Medicine* (2nd ed.). New York: Springer-Verlag, 125–40.

Bugliosi, T., Meloy, T., & Vukov, L. (1990). Acute abdominal pain in the elderly. *Annals of Emergency Medicine, 19,* 1383–6.

Butler, M. (1991). Geriatric rehabilitation nursing. *Rehabilitation Nursing, 16,* 318–21.

Byrd, S., Taylor, K., & Altmiller, R. (1987). Pain management practices in a home care hospice program. *American Journal of Hospice Care,* Nov./Dec. 21–9.

Cartwright, A., Hockey, L., & Anderson, J.L. (1973). *Life before Death.* Boston: Routledge & Kegan Paul.

Chappell, N., Strain, L., & Blandford, A. (1986). *Aging and Health Care: A Social Perspective.* Canada: Holt, Rinehart & Winston.

Clinch, D., Banerjee, A., & Ostrick, G. (1984). Absence of abdominal pain in elderly patients with peptic ulcers. *Age and Ageing, 13,* 120.

Crook, J., Rideout, E., & Browne, G. (1984). The prevalence of pain complaints in a general population. *Pain, 18,* 299–314.

Demlow, L.L., Liang, M.H., Eaton, H.M. (1986). Impact of chronic arthritis in the elderly. *Clinics in Rheumatic Diseases, 12,* 329–35.

Dobratz, M., Burns, K., & Oden, R. (1987). Pain in home hospice patients: An exploratory descriptive study. *Hospice Journal, 5,* 117–33.

Ferrell, B.A., Ferrell, B.R., & Osterwell, D. (1990). Pain in the nursing home. *Journal of the American Geriatric Society, 34,* 409–14.

Foley, K.M. (1985). The treatment of cancer pain. *New England Journal of Medicine, 113,* 84–95.

Gamsa, A. (1990), Is emotional disturbance a precipitator or consequence of chronic pain? *Pain, 4,* 138–45.

Greenwald, H.P., Bonica, J.J., & Bergner, M. (1987). The prevalence of pain in four cancers. *Cancer, 60,* 2563–9.

Haley, W.E., & Dafoe, J.J. (1986). Assessment and management of pain in the elderly. *Clinical Gerontologist, 5,* 435–55.

Harkins, S.W. (1988). Pain in the elderly. In: R. Dubner, G.G. Gebhart, & M.R. Bond (Eds.), *Pain Research and Clinical Management,* vol. 3. Amsterdam: Elsevier.

Harkins, S.W., & Chapman, C.R. (1977). Age and sex differences in pain perception. In D.J. Anderson & B. Matthews (Eds.), *Pain in the Trigeminal Region.* Amsterdam: Elsevier, 435–41.

Harkins, S.W., Kwentus, J., & Price, D. (1984). Pain and the elderly. In: C.

Benedetti, C. Chapman, & G. Moricca (Eds.), *Advances in Pain Research and Therapy*. New York: Raven.

Harris, L., and Associates (1985). *The Nuprin Pain Report*. New York: Louis Harris and Associates.

Herr, K., & Mobility, P. (1993). Comparison of selected pain assessment tools for use with the elderly. *Applied Nursing Research, 6,* 39–46.

Kane, R., Ouslander, J., & Abrass, I. (1989). *Essentials of Clinical Geriatrics*. New York: McGraw-Hill.

Kwentus, J.A., Harkins, S.W., Lignon, N., & Silverman, J.J. (1985). Current concepts of geriatric pain and its treatment. *Geriatrics, 40,* 48–57.

Liebeskind, J.C., & Melzack, R. (1987). The international pain foundation: Meeting a need for education in pain management. *Pain, 30,* 1.

Lipton, R., Pfeffer, D., Newman, L., & Soloman, S. (1993). Headaches in the elderly. *Journal of Pain and Symptom Management, 8,* 87–97.

MacDonald, S., Baillie, J., Willian, B., & Ballantyne, D. (1983). Coronary care in the elderly. *Age and Ageing, 12,* 17–60.

Magni, J., Schtano, F., & Deleo, D. (1985). Pain as a symptom in elderly depressed patients: Relationship to diagnostic sub-groups. *European Archives of Psychiatry and Neurological Services, 235,* 143–5.

Mansfield, J., & Marx, M. (1993). Pain and depression in the nursing home: Corroborating results. *Journals of Gerontolgoy: Psychological Sciences, 48,* 96–7.

Melding, P. (1992). Psychological aspects of chronic pain and the elderly. *International Association for the Study of Pain Newsletter,* Jan./Feb., 2–4.

Mor, V. (1987). *Hospice Care Systems: Structure, Process, Costs, and Outcomes*. New York: Springer-Verlag.

Morris, J.N., Mor, V., Goldberg, R.J., Sherwood, S., Greer, D.S., & Hiris, J. (1986a). The effect of treatment setting and patient characteristics on pain in terminal cancer patients. *Journal of Chronic Disease, 39,* 27–35.

Morris, J.N., Suissa, S., Sherwood, S., Wright, S.M., & Greer, D. (1986b). Last days: A study of the quality of life of terminally ill cancer patients. *Journal of Chronic Disease, 39,* 47-62.

Moss, M., Lawton, M., & Glicksman, A. (1991). The role of pain in the last year of life of older persons. *Journal of Gerontology, 42,* 51–7.

Newman, L., Lipton, R., & Solomon, S. (1991). The hypnic headache syndrome. In F.C. Rose, (Ed.), *New Advances in Headache Research* (2nd ed.). Great Britain: Smith-Gordon.

Osburn, R., Simmons Tropea, D., & Schwenger, C. (1986). Health Status and Health Services for Elderly Canadians. The Programme in Gerontology, University of Toronto.

Parmelee, P., Katz, I.R., & Lawton, M.P. (1991). The relation of pain to depression among institutionalized aged. *Journals of Gerontology: Psychological Sciences,* *46,* P15–P21.

Raskin, M.N. (1988). *Headache* (2nd ed.). New York: Churchill-Livingston.

Romano, J.M., & Turner, J.A. (1985). Chronic pain and depression: Does the evidence support a relationship? *Psychological Bulletin, 97,* 18–34.

Roy, R., & Thomas, M. (1986). Survey of chronic pain in an elderly population. *Canadian Family Physician, 32,* 513–16.

Roy, R., Thomas, M., & Matas, M. (1984). Chronic pain and depression: A review. *Comprehensive Psychiatry, 25,* 96–105.

Sheridan, M.S. (1992) *Pain in America.* Tuscaloosa, Alabama: University of Alabama Press.

Sloan, J.P. (1992). Prescribing strategies for the frail elderly. *Canadian Family Physician, 38,* 2422–8.

Solomon, G., Kunkel, R., & Frame, J. (1990). Demographics of headache in elderly patients. *Headache, 30,* 273–6.

Sorkin, B., Rudy, T., Hanlon, R., Turk, D., & Stieg, R. (1990). Chronic pain in old and young patients: Differences appear less important than similarities. *Journal of Gerontology, 45,* 64–8.

Statistics Canada (1990). *A Portrait of Seniors in Canada.* Ottawa: Minister of Supplies and Services Canada.

Stelian, J., Gil, I., Habot, B., Rosenthal, M., Abramovici, J., Kutok, N., & Khakit, A. (1992). Improvement of pain and disability in elderly patients with degenerative arthritis of the knee treated with narrow band light therapy. *Journal of the American Geriatrics Society, 40,* 23–6.

Stewart, W., Lipton, R., Celentano, D., & Reed, M. (1992). Prevalence of migraine headache in the United States. *Journal of the American Medical Association, 267,* 64–9.

Thienhaus, O.J. (1989). Pain in the elderly. In K.M. Foley and R.M. Payne (Eds.), *Current Therapy of Pain.* Toronto: B.C. Decker, 82–9.

Thomas, M., & Roy, R. (1988). Age and pain: A comparative study of the younger and older elderly. *Journal of Pain Management, 1,* 174–9.

Tunks, E., (1988). Determining the causes of neurologic pain in the elderly. *Geriatrics,* 21–9.

Tunks, E., (1990). Is there a chronic pain syndrome? In: Lipton (Eds.) *Advances in Pain Research and Therapy* (13th ed.). New York: Raven Press, 257–66.

Turk, D.C., & Rudy, T.E. (1986). Assessment of cognitive factors in chronic pain: A worthwhile enterprise? *Journal of Consulting and Clinical Psychology, 54,* 760–8.

Twycross, R.G., & Lack, S.A. (1983). *Symptom Control in Advanced Cancer: Pain Relief.* London: Pitman.

Valkenburg, H. (1988). Epidemiologic considerations of the geriatric population. *Gerontology, 34* (suppl.), 2–10.

Van Der Does, A.J. (1989). Patients and nurses rating of pain and anxiety during burn wound care. *Pain, 39,* 95.

Vanharanta, H., Sachs, B., Ohnmeiss, M., & April, C. (1989). Pain provocation and disc deterioration by age. *Spine, 14,* 420–3.

Van Korff., Dworkin, S.F., Le Resche, L., & Kruger, A. (1988). An epidemiologic comparison of pain complaints. *Pain, 32,* 173–83.

Wade, I., Morin, C., Schwartz, S., & Walton, E. *Sleep and Emotional Disturbance in Chronic Pain Patients.* Paper presented at the annual meeting of the Association for Advancement of Behaviour Therapy. Washington, DC.

Warren, R.W., & O'Brien, S.J. (1989). Shoulder pain in the geriatric patient: Approaches to senior care. *Orthopedic Review, 18,* 129–35.

Williamson, G.M., & Schultz, R. (1992). Pain, activity restriction, and symptoms of depression among community-residing elderly adults. *Journal of Gerontology, 47,* 367–72.

Witte, M. (1989). Pain control. *Journal of Gerontological Nursing, 15,* 32–7.

2

Attitudes, Beliefs, and Illness Behaviour

ANDREW COOK and RANJAN ROY

In this chapter we seek to explore some of the very complex issues that in our judgment profoundly influence the behaviour of individuals afflicted by inexplicable pain. It is the inexplicability of the chronic pain condition that fuels the mystique of medicine and causes further confusion in the minds of those who have to live with the vicissitudes of this affliction. The literature on the attitudes, beliefs, and illness behaviour of the elderly with chronic benign pain is virtually non-existent. Many of the issues, however, have been examined in relation to arthritis (a prototype for chronic pain) in the elderly. Additionally, a great deal of the literature is of a non-clinical nature. Based on our experience of working with older patients with chronic pain, we have endeavoured to articulate in this chapter the clinical ramifications and significance of their belief systems. We have also addressed, albeit briefly, some of the problems of clashing belief systems between patients and their physicians.

Anyone who has had even a passing experience of working with pain clinic patients, young or old, is immediately struck by the confusion of these patients as they begin to comprehend the absence of a coherent explanation for their pain. The cause is unknown and the cure elusive. Those who may be fortunate enough to have a diagnosis are frustrated by their lack of progress, and again their belief in the magic of modern medicine is strained. Under such circumstances, it is only natural that they will experience considerable dismay and attempt to reconstruct their beliefs (though many refuse to do so) about the organic etiology of pain.

For the past several years one of us (RR) has routinely asked newly admitted patients at the pain clinic about their 'theory' of the causes of their pain. The most common reply is 'I don't know,' followed by 'Maybe they haven't really tried to find out what's wrong with me.' The implication is that most patients are committed to finding a plausible biomedical explanation that provides some vindication for their pain and suffering, which is not always believed by all. Indeed, the influence of the biomedical model in shaping their belief system about cause and treatment is almost unqualified.

Attitudes of elderly chronic pain sufferers seem to vary somewhat with the severity of the problem. It has been observed that healthy elderly persons living in the community tend to minimize their pain problems, accept pain as very much a part of growing old, and continue to enjoy a very full life (Cook and Thomas, 1994; Roy and Thomas, 1987). In a similar vein Schorr, Farnham, and Ervin (1991) in their study of sixty women (64 per cent admitted to one chronic illness), age sixty-five to ninety-three years, found that most of the women perceived themselves to be in control of their daily activities with a low level of anxiety about death. In addition, the phenomenon of powerlessness 'was found to be minimal.' In contrast, in a clinical population of elderly pain clinic patients in Manchester, England, the patients manifested rather similar attitudes and belief systems as their younger counterparts (Roy, Thomas, and Berger, 1990). For example, the elderly patients were more inclined to adopt a somatic rather than psychological view of their pain, and on the Illness Behavior Questionnaire (Pilowsky, Murrel, and Gordon, 1975) their attitudes were indicative of psychological distress. However, a noteworthy fact is that pain is often less of a problem for older than younger patients for the same conditions. Prohaska, Leventhal, Leventhal, and Keller (1985) reported that older people were less likely to interpret pain symptoms as a sign of illness than were younger respondents. Similarly, Deal and associates (1985) also found that older persons with rheumatoid arthritis had fewer symptoms than younger patients (see Chapter 4).

Belgrave (1990) examined the hypothesis of illness as a stigmatizing deviance in a group of twenty-nine elderly persons with diagnosed chronic illnesses and found that 'in the presence of a named chronic disease and concrete physical problems, additional factors come to play ... She was likely to define her life in terms other than sickness.' Because chronic illness is almost anticipated by the elderly, it reduces the potential for stigma. In the absence of clear diagnosis, the chronic pain population is more vulnerable to feeling stigmatized. Yet stigmatization is less of a problem for the elderly chronic pain patient as he or she is more likely than not to have a diagnosis. However, there is another source of stigma for these individuals as their symptoms are often viewed as exaggerated, which is not an uncommon reason for their referral to the pain clinic. A seemingly disabled woman in her late seventies, confined to a wheelchair and with a history of osteoarthritis, was referred to the pain clinic for her 'unresponsiveness to therapy' and 'her tendency to exaggerate her problems and obstreperous attitude.' Her hostility to the medical profession, the root of which was her doctor's unwillingness to take her complaints seriously, was boundless. She indeed felt stigmatized.

Explanation for illness incorporates both enduring popular beliefs and deep faith in biomedical causes. For the chronic pain patient the popular beliefs and the dominant medical beliefs often merge, the reason being that pain is universally viewed as a signal for an underlying physical problem. The fact that chronic pain does not serve that purpose poses a major challenge to the patient's belief systems. In the absence of a convincing 'medical' explanation for pain, what are they to believe? The alternative, psychogenic pain (equated with madness), is unacceptable and frequently, incomprehensible.

Regardless of personal and popular belief systems, the very absence of any discernible cause or even a name for their condition creates a different order of patients' beliefs, the principal one being that the patients themselves are not believed or that their problems are met with incredulity (clear causes for stigma). This particular perception shared by many chronic pain patients is not without foundation. These patients are often mislabelled. The medical community tends to react negatively to its inability to establish plausible cause for the discrepancy between existing pathology and the patient's complaints. The belief that pain in the absence of organic cause is either improbable or psychiatric is often conveyed to the pain patient, which poses a further threat to the patient's own belief that pain is inevitably a signal for physical illness. Many patients at this point question their sanity. 'Is the pain in my head?' or 'Am I imagining this pain?' are questions fielded almost every day by pain clinic clinicians. These questions are clear indicators of the patient's belief system about the nature of her pain being placed under incredible strain. Patients run the risk of being labelled as showing signs of 'somatic delusion' or 'somatic preoccupation' when they reject the medical view of lack of physical evidence for the pain.

Is it conceivable that the belief system of the *physicians* is put to test in the face of severe pain complaints and the virtual absence of organic cause? Indeed, there is evidence that under such a circumstance, the physicians are likely to invoke 'malingering' as a possible explanation. In a survey of orthopaedic and neurosurgeons in six areas of the United States, Leavitt and Sweet (1986) found that exaggeration of symptoms and incongruity between patient's complaint and objective medical finding were the two dimensions employed by physicians to diagnose malingering. On the basis of these two attributes a significant majority of patients, young or old, male or female, attending a pain clinic would qualify as malingerers. Malingering was seen as a relatively common phenomenon by 20 per cent of the respondents. When the belief system of one group (chronic pain patients) is challenged by another (health care professionals) conflict and distrust is a predictable outcome. Such breakdown of the belief systems can give rise to self-doubt, questions about one's sanity, and even name-calling.

A sixty-seven-year-old woman with a short history of headache was told by her physician, following a neurological examination, 'We cannot find anything wrong with you. Do you know that older people usually don't get headaches?' The message was that not only was there nothing wrong with her, but she should not be having this particular problem. This patient's clinical presentation confirmed the physician's own beliefs, that is, absence of positive findings and exaggerated symptoms equal malingering. With a different set of beliefs, however, the physician could have conveyed a different message, such as 'thank goodness you don't have an aneurysm or a tumour [thus addressing the patient's major fear], but perhaps you have been under some stress of late?' Or the message commonly conveyed by pain clinic clinicians, namely, 'We don't know exactly the cause of your pain, but we are very concerned that it is causing you so much suffering. We are going to try and help you. Thankfully, there is nothing life-threatening here.' Either of the last two statements would have posed less of a threat to the patient's own beliefs and given her an opportunity to develop an alternative view(s) about the cause and meaning of her head pain.

The point is that the existing literature on the belief systems of patients has not adequately examined the dilemma of people whose medical problems are not amenable to diagnosis and treatment. In contrast, older people offer a variety of folk as well as 'scientific' explanations about the causes of arthritis. Elder (1973) noted that the uncertain etiology of arthritis has created a fertile field for 'the development of ideas derived from empirical experience and non-scientific beliefs about body-functioning.' She found that the belief system was influenced by social class as well as gender. Upper-class individuals attributed the disease to heredity or ageing, or declared ignorance of the cause. Lower-class persons more readily invoked exposure to cold or water and working conditions. Self-blame and magical thinking, such as the illness being a form of punishment, were also evident in the lower classes.

Magical thinking and self-blame in the older chronic pain population have not been systematically studied. This type of thinking may be less of a problem for the elderly pain patients as, more often than not, their pain is related to specific disorders. One investigation with the elderly patients attending a pain clinic found that every subject had a medicial diagnosis (Roy et al., 1990). Nevertheless, self-blame is periodically observed in this population, an explanation for which is not uncommonly an underlying depression rather than an enduring belief system. A sixty-eight-year-old retired executive firmly believed that his headache was the result of over-work which had caused him to neglect his wife who was slowly going blind because of diabetes. This man responded to psychotherapy and antidepressant medication.

Segall and Chappell (1991) in their investigation of beliefs about illness in the elderly concluded that health beliefs 'were not strongly associated with the age of the respondents.' Furthermore, scientific and lay beliefs often coexisted in the same social setting, and the lay community did not subscribe to some highly sophisticated belief system. In other words, 'the health beliefs held by these older adults about the meaning and management of their chronic illness do not seem to constitute a highly organized belief system.' This lack of organization manifests itself in a curious manner in the behaviour of pain clinic patients. While their belief in the physical origin of the pain problem is unequivocal, they are often willing to undergo any treatment 'as long as it helps with the pain.' This willingness enables the patients to engage in a variety of psychological interventions. Psychological treatment is not seen by them as somehow paradoxical to their biomedical understanding about the cause of pain which may have its genesis, for example, in a work-related accident.

A man in his early seventies with a diagnosis of herpes zoster was persuaded to engage in couple therapy (see Chapter 6 for detailed discussion of this case) once evidence was obtained that (a) he was capable of a higher level of functioning and (b) his wife was actively reinforcing his pain behaviours. Admittedly, it took much effort to convince him and even more to convince his wife, but they grudgingly agreed to couple therapy, with considerable benefit to the patient. The source of their resistance to treatment was their combined view that nothing was wrong in their marriage, with which the therapist concurred. However, once the purpose of the intervention, namely, to improve the patient's functional status was explained, their resistance declined. They did not seriously question the relevance of couple therapy to improve the patient's functioning. Their behaviour confirmed Segall and Chappell's proposition that highly organized belief systems are uncommon, as well as the notion that patients are likely to set aside their convictions to try 'anything that might help.'

In this section a position has been developed that the dominant belief system observed in the pain clinic population is influenced by the prevailing biomedical explanation of disease. Patients feel stigmatized, in large measure, because their complaints of 'physical' pain are discredited by the medical profession. When asked about their belief about the 'cause' of their pain, the answer is almost invariably an expression of their conviction in a physical etiology.

Fortunately, even this very firm belief is not sufficiently systematized for patients to reject psychological interventions. This paradox becomes more amenable to logic when an additional factor is considered. Pain clinic professionals have developed a high degree of sophistication in providing a multidimensional (monistic) explanation for chronic pain, which minimally begins the process of challenging the patient's rather blind subscription to the organic (dualistic) view of the pain. This softening of attitude engenders a more cooperative stance to psychological treatments, the benefits of which are not readily amenable to common sense.

PATIENT–PHYSICIAN RELATIONSHIP

The beliefs and attitudes of the elderly pain patient have an important effect in shaping relationships with physicians. The patient's beliefs about her or his pain and its causes, perceptions of her or his physicians' beliefs, and her or his general attitudes towards health professionals all directly affect the relationships and their outcomes. This is clearly a reciprocal process: The physicians' beliefs, perceptions, and attitudes are equally important in determining the quality of the relationships and their outcomes. A commonly encountered popular belief is the linkage between ageing, illness, and impairment. Higher incidence of some types of illnesses and chronic conditions in the elderly (for example, arthritis) result in the belief that many, if not all, of their health problems can be attributed solely to old age. However, empirical data yield a different reality: 'Old age is not a disease and there are no diseases attributable solely to the aging process' (Hunt, 1980). Yet, this belief is thought to affect the self-image of elderly patients, the meanings they attribute to their illnesses, and the attitudes of health professionals towards these patients (Hunt, 1980; Nuttbrock, 1986).

In contrast to this portrayal, Segall and Chappell (1991) found that only 2 per cent of 190 community residents (over age fifty) with chronic health conditions attributed their illness to old age or the ageing process. This finding was consistent with the results of a previous study on attribution of illness (Blaxter, 1983). However, the tendency to associate pain with old age is greater than the association for illness in general. Despite a growing body of research showing that pain is not a natural consequence of growing old (Harkins, Kwentus, and Price, 1984), it is commonly accepted by the elderly and their families as part of the ageing process (Cook and Thomas, 1994; Ferrell, 1991; Harkins et al., 1984; Hunt, 1980; Roy and Thomas, 1987). It is not only patients or laypersons who subscribe to this belief, but also some health care professionals (Harkins, 1988). Hunt (1980) states that 'unfortunately, it is also not uncommon for the physician to errone-ously attribute his patient's symptoms to old age with disastrous delays in achievement of a correct diagnosis and initiation of appropriate therapy.' This claim has received further support in a study of elderly community residents (Cook and Thomas, 1994), where 29 per cent of respondents reported that physicians had suggested their pain was due to the ageing process. Of the forty-seven individuals who reported chronic pain prob-lems, 38 per cent stated that their physicians had made this attribution.

These clinical portrayals and research data suggest that there is consid-erable variance in the beliefs of both elderly pain patients and their physi-cians. When there is a discrepancy in beliefs between the elderly patient and her physician, how does this influence the effectiveness of the patient–physician relationship? There is a substantial research literature in support of positive outcomes related to agreement between patient and physician about the importance of various aspects of an illness and its treatment. For chronic pain, views about appropriateness of certain kinds of treatments are often closely associated with beliefs about the origins of the pain. The redeeming effects of such patient–physician agreement have been found to include positive health outcomes (Romm, Hulka, and Mayo, 1976; Starfield et al., 1979, 1981), greater conformity to prescribed treatment regimens (Davis, 1971; Geertsen, Gray, and Ward, 1973; Svarstad, 1976), and greater patient satisfaction (DiMatteo and Hays, 1980; DiMatteo, Prince, and Taranta, 1979; Larsen, 1976; Wooley, Kane, Hughes, and Wright, 1978). Despite these empirically based relationships between patient–physician concordance and positive outcomes, desirable levels of agreement are often not achieved in practice. For example, in the area of arthritis and rheu-matic diseases, several studies have reported considerable disagreement be-tween patients and their physicians about issues of treatment (Freidin, Goldman, and Cecil, 1980; Potts, Mazzuca, & Brandt, 1986; Potts, Weinberger, and Brandt, 1984). Potts and Silverman (1990) found that a sample of thirty-five fibromyalgia patients viewed many treatment issues as significantly more important than either their physicians or a sample of rheumatologist's believed them to be. The level of disagreement was greatest between the patients and the rheumatologists. The level of satisfaction among this group of patients was predictably low for all aspects of treatment.

Potts and Silverman (1990) demonstrated the potency of physician beliefs and their effects on some areas of patient outcome. The patients of physicians who viewed psychological concerns as important were found to be less depressed and anxious than were patients of physicians who attached less importance to these factors. Similarly, patients of physicians who viewed a broad range of treatment components as important were found to have experienced less sleep disturbance and less general disability. However, it is important to maintain a realistic perspective on the influence of patient–physician agreement, as it does not override all other treatment considerations. In their study of patient and physician views regarding arthritis treatment, Potts et al. (1986) found that the reduction of patients' concerns was more strongly associated with improved health status and satisfaction than was patient–physician concordance. Agreement between the patients and their physicians about the importance of various components of the treatment plan was not associated with favourable outcomes. The authors concluded: 'The concerns identified by the patient should be addressed regardless of the clinician's own views of their importance. In some instances direct action might be taken to resolve the patient's concerns ... In other cases, it might be appropriate to discuss why the patient's concern is unwarranted' (p. 132). However, it is worthy of reiteration that elderly pain patients are, in general terms, more interested in the effectiveness of *any* intervention at reducing their pain rather than in its congruency with their belief system.

Many elderly pain sufferers have negative and even contemptuous views of the health care system. These views can represent substantial barriers to treatment if not addressed by the health professional. In a study of reasons for refusal of hospitalization among elderly patients, negative perceptions of the health care system were the primary reason given by the refusers (Barry, Crescenzi, Radovsky, Kern, and Steel, 1988). These negative perceptions included previous negative experiences, fear of hospitals, and a mistrust of the medical system. Our research with community-resident elderly (Cook and Thomas, 1994) has revealed that 8 per cent of individuals with chronic pain reported that physicians were inattentive to their pain complaints, while an additional 18 per cent reported that physicians were attentive but not helpful in dealing with their problems. These types of perceptions exert considerable power over the elderly patient's expectations of treatment and his or her interactions with health care professionals. By inquiring about the patient's attitudes and expectations, the physician can address these types of concerns and avoid perceptual obstacles to treatment.

The attitudes of health care professionals towards geriatric patients can have a substantial impact on treatment outcomes, and consequently this has been an area of considerable research interest (e.g., Ahmed, Kraft, and Porter, 1986; Cyrus-Lutz and Gaitz, 1972; Wolk and Wolk, 1971). Findings have indicated that attitudes differ among different groups of health care professionals (Ahmed et al., 1986; Belgrave, Lavin, Breslau, and Haug, 1982). For example, in their study of attitudinal differences between three groups of health professionals, Ahmed et al. (1986) found that surgeons had significantly more negative attitudes than psychiatrists or internists regarding the difficulty of obtaining a history from a geriatric patient. This type of belief has obvious implications for the patient–physician relationship. The health care professional should strive to be aware of his or her stereotypes and biases regarding the elderly pain patient – and remain open to new or unexpected explanations or methods of intervention.

HEALTH SERVICE UTILIZATION

Analogous to the assumed linkage between ageing and health problems is the belief that use of health services increases with age and that the elderly are disproportionately heavy users of health care systems. Research has failed to support these claims, revealing that age alone is not a reliable predictor of health service utilization (Barer, Evans, Hertzman, and Lomas, 1987; Haug 1981; Segall, 1987; Segall and Chappell, 1989; Wolinsky, Coe, Miller, Prendergast, Creel, and Chavez, 1983), and that a small proportion of the elderly account for a disproportionately large volume of utilization (Roos and Shapiro, 1981; Strain, 1991). Other studies have suggested that within the elderly population age differences in service use may be significant (Rivnyak, Wan, Stegall, Jacobs, and Li, 1989; Ward,1977; Wolinsky, Mosely, and Coe, 1986). These findings have directed attention to the question: What factors determine the use of health services by the elderly? Understanding the factors that affect or determine utilization behaviour in the elderly is far from complete (Coulton and Frost, 1982; Roos and Shapiro, 1981; Wolinsky et al., 1986). Variables that have been identified as significant correlates of utilization behaviour include sex, race, socioeconomic status, social networks, knowledge of available services, perceived health status, transportation barriers, marital status, cost factors, psychological distress, chronic health problems, and physical dysfunction (Cafferata, 1987;

Coulton and Frost, 1982; McCaslin, 1988; Rivnyak et al., 1989; Ward, 1977). Although the multiplicity of factors involved in health service utilization behaviour has been emphasized in much of the literature, there is a growing consensus that need for services, including perceived need and physical dysfunction, is the most important determining factor (Coulton and Frost, 1982; Rivnyak et al., 1989; Segall and Chappell, 1989; Strain, 1990, 1991; Wolinsky et al., 1983).

Despite the facts that pain is a typical warning sign of pathology and that it clearly plays an important role in perceptions of health status, its relationship to health service utilization has received little research attention. A British study that investigated self-reported morbidity and its relationship to physician visits in 1,145 adults over sixteen years of age considered the role of pain (Bucquet and Curtis, 1986). Results indicated that 'physical symptoms of pain' was one of four morbidity dimensions significantly associated with medical consultation (along with emotions, isolation, and immobility). The authors noted that respondents reporting pain or physical immobility were almost twice as likely to have consulted their physician in the past two weeks as those not reporting these symptoms. Age comparisons for this relationship were not reported, but pain and consultation rates across three age groups (sixteen to forty-four, forty-five to sixty-four, over sixty-five) indicated that medical consultation rates did not differ significantly with age. The prevalence of pain, however, was significantly affected by age, increasing from the younger to older age groups.

Elderly individuals living in the community rely on themselves as much as on formal health services for dealing with chronic pain (Cook and Thomas, 1994). The contribution of various health and demographic variables to an understanding of health service utilization was investigated in a sample of 112 elderly community residents, ages sixty-six through ninety-one (mean age, seventy-five years). Consistent with prior research, perceived health, chronic health conditions, and functional disability accounted for the majority of explained variance in health service use. Controlling for these three health dimensions, pain failed to make an incremental contribution to explaining physician visits, days in hospital, and overall health service use among these elderly individuals. The most common coping style for those afflicted with chronic pain was a combination of analgesics and accepting mild pain as part of their daily lives. Substantial relief was obtained by many of these individuals through this combination of medical intervention and attitudinal factors. As would be expected, arthritis was a major source of chronic pain among this sample, affecting 95 per cent of those reporting chronic pain.

Although pain was not a significant factor in the multivariate statistical models in this study, it is important to note that the pain variable was significantly related to both physician visits and overall health service use. That is, elderly individuals reporting more frequent and severe pain tended to be heavier users of these services. However, pain did not provide any incremental information to the understanding of service use because it was also significantly intercorrelated with the traditional measures of health status (perceived health, chronic conditions, and functional disability). Self-reported pain, like these other health variables, is largely a reflection of an individual's perceived health status, and therefore it can more appropriately be regarded as a measure of demand rather than need for health services (Wolinsky and Arnold, 1988).

The combined quantitative and qualitative data from this study confirm the common experience of the health care professional who works with geriatric patients. The majority of elderly chronic pain sufferers accept their pain as part of life and/or growing old, and this acceptance in conjunction with the use of analgesics makes it possible for them to manage their pain quite successfully. Physicians, pharmacists, and other health service providers render assistance as required and for any new problems that arise. Many of these elderly individuals report having grown accustomed to regular mild-to-moderate pain. This process of 'habituation' to pain after many decades of pain experiences is consistent with findings that the elderly report less pain than do young adults (Harris and Associates, 1985; Roy, Thomas, and Makarenko, 1989; see Chapters 3 and 4).

SELF-MANAGEMENT OF CHRONIC ILLNESS AND THE USE OF
INFORMAL RESOURCES

In addition to making use of the available formal health care services, the elderly are inevitably forced to rely on themselves for daily management of chronic illness and pain. Many elderly individuals are able to successfully develop and employ effective routines for managing their illnesses. Others are less fortunate. Regimen management, including tasks to control or monitor symptoms, restore normal body functioning, control disease processes, prevent or reverse crises, promote healing, and maintain life, can be very problematic for elderly individuals. These regimens are sometimes exhausting and complex and can affect the patient's quantity and quality of life (Corbin and Strauss, 1985).

It has been suggested that there is a core of self-management tasks common to all forms of chronic illness (Clark et al., 1991). This commonality includes such activities as monitoring certain indicators associated with the illness and taking appropriate steps in the event of monitored levels moving outside of acceptable limits. For the elderly pain patient, the most common elements of self-management regimens are self-monitoring of pain levels, taking analgesics on a scheduled or as-needed basis, doing recommended physical exercises and/or maintaining suggested activity levels, avoiding problematic activities, employing relaxation strategies, and making the necessary arrangements for daily chores that cannot be completed because of excessive pain. The life context in which these tasks must be completed is typically quite different for the elderly individual than for younger patients (Clark et al., 1991). Family structure, living arrangements, loss of peers, and other factors can greatly affect the availability of social support. In addition to directly increasing the burden of completing daily regimen tasks, inadequate levels of social support can negatively affect psychological and physical health status (Goodenow, Reisine, and Grady, 1990; Kruse and Lehr, 1989; Lambert, Lambert, Klipple, and Mewshaw, 1990; Patrick, Morgan, and Charlton, 1986; Roberto, 1988; Weinberger, Hiner, and Tierney, 1986).

The social support network of the elderly pain patient provides an informal resource for consultation regarding health concerns. In a study of seventy-eight arthritic elderly individuals, Strain (1990) found that virtually all consulted at least one family member or friend about their affliction on a regular basis. This lay consultation included exchanging facts and medical or non-medical advice or sometimes only a reporting of the current condition. Consultations were reported for occasions prior to visiting health professionals, following such visits, and also at times when there was no use of formal health services. Spouses were the most common consultants, followed by children and friends.

Other research has suggested that the elderly rely on their peers and counterparts for this type of consultation and avoid discussions with their children (Furstenberg, 1985). This finding was interpreted in terms of several possible benefits from consultations with age peers: (a) meeting social needs, (b) providing an equalized exchange and opportunity to compare problems, and (c) encountering a greater familiarity with illness and afflictions of the elderly among this peer group.

Lay consultation is clearly an important part of self-management of chronic illness by the elderly. In working with the elderly pain patient, it is worthwhile to inquire about informal resources and the social support network. If adequate resources exist, then the patient can be encouraged to turn to these individuals for required support. A lack of adequate social support can perhaps be mitigated by more frequent consultation with health professionals, and opportunities for participation in educational/support groups can be explored.

SUMMARY

The central pursuit for elderly, as for all, chronic pain sufferers is to obtain relief from pain. When that objective is thwarted, beliefs about the cause and cure are severely strained. Some elderly people show considerable courage and endurance in tolerating, day to day, what are sometimes severe aches and pains, and they have an almost fatalistic attitude towards living with pain. In this respect they are fundamentally different from the young pain sufferers who seek immediate relief. Unfortunately, many health care professionals and certainly the general population also view pain in old age as inevitable. Because psychogenic pain is relatively uncommon in the elderly, they do not always have the benefit of careful psychosocial and psychiatric assessment and treatment.

The writing of this chapter presented some interesting challenges. The literature relevant to the topic was sparse and often only indirectly related. In addition, clinical as opposed to sociological literature was even less evident. Hence, much of the chapter is based on inferences, extrapolations, and the authors' experiences of working with elderly chronic pain patients. Despite these shortcomings, some of the issues discussed here merit special mention.

First and foremost, young or old, male or female, patients with intractable problems of chronic pain want to be believed about their pain and suffering in an unconditional way. Second, their belief systems should be carefully explored and alternative views offered in a manner that does not discredit their viewpoint. Third, the health care professionals should be aware of their own beliefs and prejudices and be very cautious not to condemn beliefs that are contrary to their own. Fourth, as has been demonstrated, alternative viewpoints are always available, and, when humanely offered, patients are quite willing to accept the alternatives. Depression and other psychological conditions can and do complicate the pain presentation in the elderly, as they seem to do with greater frequency among younger patients. Finally, health care professionals need to be more aware of the impact their statements have on their patients. Most patients do not subscribe to unalterable beliefs about the causes and cures of their pain problems. Proper explanation and gentle persuasion are often enough to achieve cooperation in treatment.

REFERENCES

Ahmed, S.M., Kraft, I.A., & Porter, D.M. (1986). Attitudes of different professional groups toward geriatric patients. *Gerontology and Geriatrics Education, 6*, 77–86.

Barer, M.L., Evans, R.G., Hertzman, C., & Lomas, J. (1987). Aging and health care utilization: New evidence on old fallacies. *Social Science and Medicine, 24*, 851–62.

Barry, P.P., Crescenzi, C.A., Radovsky, L., Kern, D.C., & Steel, K. (1988). Why elderly patients refuse hospitalization. *Journal of the American Geriatrics Society, 36*, 419–24.

Belgrave, L. (1990). The relevance of chronic illness in the everyday lives of elderly women. *Journal of Aging and Health, 2*, 475–500.

Belgrave, L.L., Lavin, B., Breslau, N., & Haug, M.R. (1982). Stereotyping of the aged by medical students. *Gerontology and Geriatrics Education, 3*, 37–44.

Blaxter, M. (1983). The cause of disease: Women talking. *Social Science and Medicine, 17*, 59–69.

Bucquet, D., & Curtis, S. (1986). Socio-demographic variation in perceived illness and the use of primary care: The value of community survey data for primary care service planning. *Social Science and Medicine, 23*, 737–44.

Cafferata, G.L. (1987). Marital status, living arrangements, and the use of health services by elderly persons. *Journal of Gerontology, 42*, 613–18.

Clark, N.M., Becker, M.H., Janz, N.K., Lorig, K., Rakowski, W., & Anderson, L. (1991). Self-management of chronic disease by older adults: A review and questions for research. *Journal of Aging and Health, 3*, 3–27.

Cook, A.J., & Thomas, M.R. (1994). Pain and the use of health services among the elderly. *Journal of Aging and Health, 6*, 155–72.

Corbin, J.M., & Strauss, A.L. (1985). Issues concerning regimen management in the home. *Ageing and Society, 5*, 249–65.

Coulton, C., & Frost, A.K. (1982). Use of social and health services by the elderly. *Journal of Health and Social Behavior, 23*, 330–9.

Cyrus-Lutz, C., & Gaitz, C.M. (1972). Psychiatrists' attitudes toward the aged and aging. *Gerontologist, 1*, 163–7.

Davis, M.S. (1971). Variation in patients' compliance with doctors' orders: Medical practice and doctor–patient interaction. *Psychiatric Medicine, 2*, 31–54.

Deal, C., Meenan D., Goldenberg, J., Anderson, R., Sack, B., Pastan, R., & Cohen, A. (1985). The clinical features of early-onset rheumatoid arthritis. *Arthritis and Rheumatism, 28*, 987–94.

DiMatteo, R.M., & Hays, R. (1980). The significance of patients' perceptions of physician conduct: A study of patient satisfaction in a family practice centre. *Journal of Community Health, 6*, 18–34.

DiMatteo, R.M., Prince, L.M., & Taranta, A. (1979). Patients' perceptions of physicians' behavior: Determinants of patient commitment to the therapeutic relationship. *Journal of Community Health, 4*, 280–90.

Elder, R. (1973). Social class and lay explanations of the etiology of arthritis. *Journal of Health and Social Behavior, 14*, 28–38.

Ferrell, B.A. (1991). Pain management in elderly people. *Journal of the American Geriatrics Society, 39*, 64–73.

Freidin, R.B., Goldman, L., & Cecil, R.R. (1980). Patient–physician concordance in problem identification in the primary care setting. *Annals of Internal Medicine, 93*, 490–3.

Furstenberg, A.L. (1985). Older people's choices of lay consultants. *Journal of Gerontological Social Work, 9*, 21–34.

Geertsen, H.R., Gray, R.M., & Ward, J.R. (1973). Patient non-compliance within the context of seeking medical care for arthritis. *Journal of Chronic Diseases, 26*, 689–98.

Goodenow, C., Reisine, S.T., & Grady, K.E. (1990). Quality of social support and associated social and psychological functioning in women with rheumatoid arthritis. *Health Psychology, 9*, 266–84.

Harkins, S.W. (1988). Issues in the study of pain and suffering in relation to age. *International Journal of Technology and Aging, 1*, 146–55.

Harkins, S.W., Kwentus, J., & Price, D.D. (1984). Pain and the elderly. In: C. Benedetti, C.R. Chapman, & G. Moricca (Eds.), *Advances in Pain Research and Therapy: vol. 7. Recent Advances in the Management of Pain*. New York: Raven, 103–21.

Harris, L., and Associates (1985). *The Nuprin Pain Report*. New York: L. Harris & Associates.

Haug, M.R. (1981). Age and medical care utilization patterns. *Journal of Gerontology, 36*, 103–11.

Hunt, T.E. (1980). Pain and the aged patient. In: W.L. Smith, H. Merskey, & S.C. Gross (Eds.), *Pain: Meaning and Management*. New York: Spectrum, 143–57.

Kruse, A., & Lehr, U. (1989). Longitudinal analysis of the developmental process in chronically ill and healthy persons: Empirical findings from the Bohn Longitudinal Study of Aging (BOLSA). *International Psychogeriatrics, 1*, 73–85.

Lambert, V.A., Lambert, C.E., Klipple, G.L., & Mewshaw, E.A. (1990). Relationships among hardiness, social support, severity of illness, and psychological well-being in women with rheumatoid arthritis. *Health Care for Women International, 11*, 159–73.

Larsen, D.E. (1976). Physician role performance and patient satisfaction. *Social Science and Medicine, 10*, 29–32.

Leavitt, F., & Sweet, B. (1986). Characteristics and frequency of malingering among patients with low back pain. *Pain, 25,* 357–64.

McCaslin, R. (1988). Reframing research on service use among the elderly: An analysis of recent findings. *Gerontologist, 28,* 592–9.

Nuttbrock, L. (1986). Socialization to the chronic sick role in later life: An interactionist view. *Research on Aging, 8,* 368–87.

Patrick, D.L., Morgan, M., & Charlton, J.R. (1986). Psychosocial support and change in the health status of physically disabled people. *Social Science and Medicine, 22,* 1347–54.

Pilowsky, I., Murrell, T.G.C., & Gordon, A. (1975). The development of a screening method for abnormal illness behaviour. *Journal of Psychosomatic Research, 23,* 203–7.

Potts, M.K., Mazzuca, S.A., & Brandt, K.D. (1986). Views of patients and physicians regarding the importance of various aspects of arthritis treatment: Correlations with health status and patient satisfaction. *Patient Education and Counseling, 8,* 125–34.

Potts, M.K., & Silverman, S.L. (1990). The importance of aspects of treatment for fibromyalgia (fibrositis): Differences between patient and physician views. *Arthritis Care and Research, 3,* 11–18.

Potts, M., Weinberger, M., & Brandt, K.D. (1984). Views of patients and providers regarding the importance of various aspects of an arthritis treatment program. *Journal of Rheumatology, 11,* 71–5.

Prohaska, T., Leventhal, A., Leventhal, H., & Keller, M. (1985). Health practices: Illness cognition in young, middle-aged, and elderly adults. *Journal of Gerontology, 40,* 569–78.

Rivnyak, M.H., Wan, T.T.H., Stegall, M.H., Jacobs, M., & Li, S. (1989). Ambulatory care use among the non-institutionalized elderly: A causal model. *Research on Aging, 11,* 292–311.

Roberto, K.A. (1988). Women with osteoporosis: The role of the family and service community. *Gerontologist, 28,* 224–8.

Romm, F.J., Hulka, B.S., & Mayo, F. (1976). Correlates of outcome in patients with congestive heart failure. *Medical Care, 14,* 765–76.

Roos, N.P., & Shapiro, E. (1981). The Manitoba longitudinal study on aging. *Medical Care, 19,* 644–57.

Roy, R., & Thomas, M.R. (1987). Pain, depression, and illness behavior in a community sample of active elderly persons: Elderly persons with and without pain: (Part II). *Clinical Journal of Pain, 3,* 207–11.

Roy, R., Thomas, M., & Berger, S. (1990). A comparative study of British and Canadian pain patients. *Clinical Journal of Pain, 6,* 276–83.

Roy, R., Thomas, M., & Makarenko, P. (1989). Memories of pain: Comparison of 'worst pain ever' experienced by senior citizens and college students. *Clinical Journal of Pain, 5*, 359–62.

Schorr, J., Farnham, R., & Ervin, S. (1991). Health patterns in aging women as expanding consciousness. *Advances in Nursing Science, 13*, 52–63.

Segall, A. (1987). Age differences in lay conceptions of health and self-care responses to illness. *Canadian Journal on Aging, 6*, 47–65.

Segall, A., & Chappell, N.L. (1989). Health care beliefs and the use of medical and social services by the elderly. In: S.J. Lewis (Ed.), *Aging and Health: Linking Research and Public Policy*. Chelsea, MI: Lewis, 129–41.

Segall, A., & Chappell, N.L. (1991). Making sense out of sickness: Lay explanations of chronic illness among older adults. *Advances in Medical Sociology, 2*, 115–33.

Starfield, B., Steinwachs, D., Morris, I., Bause, G., Siebert, S., & Westin, C. (1979). Patient–doctor agreement about problems needing follow-up visits. *Journal of the American Medical Association, 242*, 344–6.

Starfield, B., Wray, C., Hess, K., Gross, R., Birk, P., & D'Lugoff, B.C. (1981). The influence of patient–practitioner agreement on outcome of care. *American Journal of Public Health, 71*, 127–31.

Strain, L.A. (1990). Lay consultation among the elderly: Experiences with arthritis. *Journal of Aging and Health, 2*, 103–22.

Strain, L.A. (1991). Use of health services in later life: The influence of health beliefs. *Journal of Gerontology, 46*, S143–50.

Svarstad, B.L. (1976). Physician–patient communications and patient conformity with medical advice. In D. Mechanic (Ed.), *The Growth of Bureaucratic Medicine*. New York: Wiley, 222–38.

Ward, R.A. (1977). Services for older people: An integrated framework for research. *Journal of Health and Social Behavior, 18*, 61–70.

Weinberger, M., Hiner, S.L., & Tierney, W.M. (1986). Improving functional status in arthritis: The effects of social support. *Social Science and Medicine, 23*, 899–904.

Wolinsky, F.D., & Arnold, C.L. (1988). A different perspective on health and health services utilization. *Annual Review of Gerontology and Geriatrics, 8*, 71–101.

Wolinsky, F.D., Coe, R.M., Miller, D.K., Prendergast, J.M., Creel, M.J., & Chavez, M.N. (1983). Health services utilization among the non-institutionalized elderly. *Journal of Health and Social Behavior, 24*, 325–37.

Wolinsky, F. D., Mosely, R.R., & Coe, R.M. (1986). A cohort analysis of the use of health services by elderly Americans. *Journal of Health and Social Behavior, 27*, 209–19.

Wolk, R.L, & Wolk, R.B. (1971). Professional workers' attitudes toward the aged. *Journal of the American Geriatrics Society, 19*, 624–39.

Wooley, F.R., Kane, R.L., Hughes, C.C., & Wright, D.D. (1978). The effects of doctor-patient communication on satisfaction and outcome of care. *Social Science and Medicine, 12*, 123–8.

3

Pain among Healthy Elderly Individuals

MICHAEL THOMAS

In the year 1900 only 4 per cent of the North American population was over the age of sixty-five. In the 1990s approximately 15 per cent of the population will be sixty-five years or older, and by 2040 it is estimated that as much as 25 per cent of the population (ninety million individuals) in North America will be in this age range (Guralnik, Yanagashita, and Schneider, 1988). This chapter will review the literature regarding pain reported in the 'healthy elderly' population. It is of increasing importance to understand the pain experiences of the healthy elderly, because this age group constitutes the fastest growing segment of the population in industrialized countries. Individuals in this age group are increasing proportionally to the world population because of a number of factors such as: (a) improvements in medical technology; (b) new drug developments; (c) better education; (d) healthier lifestyles; (e) decreased mortality rates of infants and mothers; (f) better control of infectious diseases; and (g) wider access to medical care.

Current projections for the average life span in the United States and Canada from census data in the 1980s estimate eighty-three years for women and seventy-nine years for men. These figures represent estimated averages, which means that individuals reaching the age of sixty-five, because of the mortality that has occurred already in their cohorts, can expect to be functional well into their eighties (Melding, 1991). For the purpose of research, those over age sixty-five can be placed into three groups: the young-old (sixty-five to seventy-four years), the old-old (seventy-five to eighty-four), and the oldest-old (eighty-five and over). The oldest-old, currently 1 per cent of the population, are projected to become 5 per cent of the population by 2050. At any time a majority of the elderly are healthy and staying healthy longer, although it should be noted that the elderly as individuals have the largest range of functional differences in health status of any age group.

PROBLEMS OF DEFINITIONS

Given the large proportion of the population that falls into the elderly age range, how exactly is health defined in this group? The *Oxford English Dictionary* defines health as soundness of body or mind. The psychological and medical research literature, however, appears to define health in the elderly most frequently as the absence of diagnosable pathology. This definition of absence of illness in the research literature regarding the healthy elderly, in all probability, has contributed significantly to the common myth that ageing is synonymous with poor health and pain.

Because of gender differences in longevity, over 75 per cent of the elderly population are women. This results in some demographic distortions describing the 'healthy elderly.' Social demographics also suggest that the elderly in North America maintain 'traditional' family lifestyles as long as health allows. Approximately 80 per cent of the men between sixty-five and seventy-four are married compared with 49 per cent of the women in this age range. Elderly widowed men have a remarriage rate seven times that of widows (United States Bureau of the Census, 1986).

Ageing leads ultimately to death in the individual, but is this journey through life inevitably filled with declining health and increasing pain? Many questions related to pain in the healthy elderly remain unresolved by empirical data. Increasing numbers of the North American population of all ages are becoming more health conscious. Preliminary surveys indicate elderly individuals employ a wide range of coping mechanisms to deal with pain and illness as well as improving or maintaining their health status (Harris and Guten, 1979; Prohaska, Laventhal, Laventhal, and Keller, 1985; Leventhal and Prohaska, 1986).

The influence of psychological and social factors that account for different attitudes towards health, pain, and subsequent behaviours throughout the life span is in the early stages of investigation – or simply unknown at present (Lau, 1982; Gochman, 1985; Prohaska et al., 1985; Prohaska, Keller, Leventhal, and Leventhal, 1987). Research on psychological coping in relation to pain, illness, and health in the elderly is also limited (Haley and Dolce, 1986; Keefe and Williams, 1990; Ferrell, 1991; Fry and Wong, 1991).

AGEING AND PAIN: PHYSICAL, MENTAL, AND
PSYCHOLOGICAL INFLUENCES

Harkins (1988) in a review of the sensory literature notes that with increasing age a decline in sensitivity with many of the senses has been well documented. Current research findings confirm that physical changes may commence in some healthy individuals in their fifties and typically by the sixties the changes are quite obvious. Shifts in sensory threshold accompany decreases in reaction time, agility, physical mobility, and physical strength (Buskist and Gerbing, 1990). However, the laboratory study of pain thresholds and pain perception in relation to ageing at present has not produced consistent findings (Harkins, 1988). Pain threshold, unlike pain tolerance, can be quantitatively measured in physical units. Overall, in healthy individuals there is typically small variation (under 20 per cent) in pain thresholds as well as minimal variation (under 30 per cent) in sensitivity over the different areas of the body of an individual. In a recent study, Tucker, Andrew, Ogle, and Davison (1989) found a rapid rise in pain threshold until age twenty-five followed by a more gradual rise in pain threshold until about age seventy-five, but after age eighty the wide variability of pain thresholds eluded any general conclusions. Furthermore, this study found no sex differences in pain threshold and no significant differences in pain thresholds between subjects with pain and without pain.

If physiological measures in the healthy elderly cannot predict pain reports, then it is possible that many pain symptoms are attributable to psychological and/or social factors, or to the ageing process *per se*. Pain threshold perception by older adults is further complicated by the presence, in some individuals, of multiple health problems with vague symptoms that can affect the same areas of the body. Threshold is primarily a measure of the sensory dimension of pain. Current thinking conceptualizes pain along multiple dimensions including the psychological and social. Therefore, pain tolerance rather than pain threshold is actually more relevant both to the reporting of pain in the healthy elderly and for self-ratings of health in the elderly.

Memory and Pain

Another variable, affected by declining efficiency starting as early as the twenties for some individuals but universally manifested by the fifties, is memory. The issue of declining memory in the healthy elderly is important, because pain research with the elderly tends to consist of retrospective self-reports of illness, pain, medical treatment, and general health. This body of research becomes suspect with regard to reliability (Gilewski and Zelinski, 1986; Sunderland, Watts, Baddeley, and Harris, 1986; Roy, Thomas, and Makarenko, 1990). The loss of memory functioning associated with ageing is typically a reduction in speed of recall with some lapses in recall that are generally associated with problems in encoding or retrieving information (Poon, 1985). There are, however, data to the contrary. In a recent United States survey (n = 14,783) approximately 15 per cent of persons over the age of fifty-five complained of frequent memory problems, while 25 per cent reported they had never had memory problems. In this large sample only 23 per cent of the oldest-old (age eighty-five or over) reported having frequent memory difficulties (Cutler and Grams, 1988). In an earlier study, performance on learning and memory tasks was unrelated to age with the health variable held constant (Hulicka, 1967). Diminishing memory functioning with increasing age in the healthy elderly is less of a problem than may be popularly believed.

In a study investigating memories of worst pain in healthy elderly and young adult subjects, all subjects remembered recent pain as the most intense with the exception of a small number of elderly individuals who recalled distant past pain (childbirth) as most intense, which was speculated to have been associated with psychological trauma (Roy et al., 1990). The results from this study also indicated a shift in the experience of worst pain across life span such that young subjects reported trauma, headache, and stomach cramps as 'worst pain,' while the elderly reported chronic pain problems such as arthritis as the 'worst pain.' The study further found that rates of hospitalization were equivalent between the young and the healthy elderly group, although young and elderly were hospitalized for different health problems.

Ageing and Cognitive Functioning

Another variable that has been investigated in relation to ageing and impact on pain is intellectual functioning. Current research using appropriate mixes of longitudinal and cross-sectional research designs has found that intellectual functioning shifts with ageing in healthy individuals. The slow decline, especially in verbal functioning with ageing, in the healthy elderly, appears to have minimal influences on pain behaviours. Recent studies have found no significant age effects in cognitive strategies used for coping with chronic pain (Keefe and Williams, 1990; Fry and Wong, 1991; also see Chapter 4). Shifts in intellectual functioning as the result of ageing in the healthy elderly vary depending upon the type of cognitive function assessed. For verbal I.Q. measures (functioning most related to social/psychological aspects of pain behaviours) there are continuing increases in measured intelligence scores until after age seventy. On average the verbal functioning of healthy individuals is better when they are in their seventies than when they are in their twenties (Schaie, 1982; Schaie and Willis, 1986).

Pain and Depression

There is limited research specifically investigating psychosomatic pain complaints in the healthy elderly (see Chapter 10). This is not surprising, because less than 5 per cent of individuals aged sixty-five or older attend pain clinics where psychosomatic pain is likely to be diagnosed. However, the link between physical health, pain, and depression beyond the unhappiness that normally accompanies an illness or pain is well documented (Roy, Thomas, and Matas, 1984; Parmelee, Katz, and Lawton, 1989).

Depressive behaviours are frequently present in the healthy elderly, although clinical depression is unusual (Roy and Thomas, 1988). In a study by Parmelee, Katz, and Lawton (1991) with a sample of institutionalized elderly people who did not have chronic pain, individuals diagnosed with major depression reported more intense pain and a greater number of localized pain locations than did mildly depressed or non-depressed individuals. This study is of interest in regard to pain in the healthy elderly because it controlled statistically for functional disability and health status. With disability and health controlled for, no relationship between age and pain intensity or number of localized complaints was found, although there were sex differences, with women reporting more intensity and more pain locations. Location of pain was related to depression except in the case of headaches or joint pains. These data seem to suggest that in the elderly, neither physical infirmity nor age is the factor underlying the relationship between depression and pain complaints.

There are many plausible explanations for the relationship between pain and depression in the elderly. Depression may psychologically sensitize individuals to pain so that their psychological reactions to physical discomfort become intensified to an interpretation of pain, according to Waddell (1987), who even argues that the physical stimulus that triggers a painful sensation may across time become less salient, and emotional distress such as depression becomes responsible in sustaining the psychological experience of pain. This proposition requires further validation.

Gender and Pain

Gender differences in pain reports in the healthy elderly are another area of interest. The cognitive processes occurring during depression have been found to be similar to the cognitive processes when experiencing pain (Peterson and Seligman, 1984). The relationship between depressive cognitive processes and cognitive processes present during experiences of pain is consistent with the findings that women have more reported depression as well as pain complaints than do men throughout their lives, although this phenomenon may reflect reporting bias, because there is also evidence that women generally are depicted as physically and psychologically less healthy than men (Kaplan, Barell, and Lusky, 1988).

REPORTED PAIN EXPERIENCES IN THE ELDERLY

There are consistent data indicating high correlations between reported pain experiences and the elderly (over sixty-five years). Brody, Kleban, and Moles (1983) reported that 73 per cent of an elderly population noted pain of some type during a twenty-four-hour period. Demlow, Laing, and Eaton (1986) reported 80 per cent of an elderly population had some form of rheumatic pain. Roy and Thomas (1986, 1987) found that 70 per cent of a healthy elderly population complained of some type of pain, and 83 per cent of an elderly nursing home population reported pain. Previous studies of residents in nursing homes have found up to 85 per cent reporting pain on a more or less continuous basis. However, a nursing population is not a representative sample of the elderly population.

It is likely that with ageing the prevalence of pain ranges somewhere between 35 and 85 per cent in the elderly population at large. To date only one study has directly compared reported pain frequencies and locations between a clinical pain patient sample with a 'healthy' sample in the elderly population (Roy, Thomas, and Berger, 1990). The clinical pain elderly group and the healthy elderly group were matched on demographic variables such that there were no significant differences on any factors except for income level. The clinical pain group reported a lower average income.

Table 1 shows the reported frequencies of the most common pain locations. The data indicated that the frequency of joint pain in the 'healthy' elderly was similar to the frequency of joint pain in the clinical pain elderly group, while the reported frequency of back pain was higher in the clinical pain elderly group. There was a large mean difference between the two

Table 1. Reported frequencies of the most common pain locations

Pain variables	Healthy elderly (N = 143)	Clinical pain (N = 46)
Location		
Back (%)	40.0	57.8*
Joint (%)	35.5	37.8
Mean duration (years)	15.2	7.45
Mean pain level	2.4	6.90**

*Not significant; ** $p < 0.0001$

elderly groups in duration of pain, but the difference was non-significant because of the extreme variability in reported durations in the two groups. Paradoxically, the 'healthy' elderly group reported a mean pain duration greater than the clinical pain elderly group did. The clinical pain group reported significantly higher pain intensity, appeared more depressed, and scored higher on the Illness Behavior Questionnaire – indicating more psychological dysfunction. Finally, the use of medication for pain was significantly higher in the clinical pain elderly group.

It is critical that in any attempt to improve understanding of the relationship between age and pain, any uniformity in the incidence of pain, living styles, or background characteristics for individuals whose ages span at least a twenty-year interval (sixty-five to eight-five) cannot be assumed. One variable that has an impact on research in the healthy elderly group is the relationship between the death rate in the elderly and illness and pain. The elderly who survive and move from the youngest-old to oldest-old status represent a selected healthier sample than a less selected sample (based on survival) of younger-old. Second, it would seem that the elderly who typically participate in non-clinical pain research are healthier than the general elderly population. Very few studies have compared health and pain variables between youngest-old, old-old, and oldest-old subjects, as well as made a comparison with subjects from other age groups. Those that have reported directly on age and pain have used inappropriate statistical methods such as intermixing of continuous and discrete data during analysis. Finally, one of the most critical variables in researching pain in the elderly, namely, health status, is typically not controlled statistically or through subject selection techniques.

Healthy Elderly with and without Pain

In a group of studies (Thomas and Roy, 1988; Thomas, Roy, and Makarenko, 1989; Roy and Thomas, 1987, 1988, 1989) involving elderly non-clinical pain populations, social and psychological factors were investigated. Roy and Thomas (1987, 1988) drew a random sample from an elderly population living in the community who did not have illness or health problems severe enough to require hospitalization during the previous six months. Thus, using a negative definition of exclusion, this group was classified as healthy elderly, because they were socially and physically functional. In this study the healthy elderly with and without pain complaints were compared.

The relationship between pain and age for this elderly sample is presented in Table 2.

On the basis of this study, pain in the elderly appears common, approximately 70 per cent reported some type of current pain, yet these same individuals did not report the presence of social or physical disability caused by pain. This result reflects attitudes towards pain best described by comments from individual elderly subjects that 'having to live with pain was in the same order as not being able to run as they did when they were younger, it was just a matter of accepting the fact of aging.'

In another study Thomas and Roy (1988) found 73 per cent of a healthy elderly sample of subjects reported chronic pain. For the sixties age group, 81 per cent reported pain for all locations, and for the eighties age group, only 64 per cent reported pain for all body locations. The pain and age relationship was non-significant but demonstrated a strong trend for older elderly to report less pain than the younger elderly. Sex and age breakdown of additional pain data indicated that for the women in the sixties group who reported chronic pain the mean duration was 12.5 years, furthermore 49 per cent of the women reported taking medication, while only 6 per cent reported having ever attended a pain clinic. In comparison the women in the eighties group who reported chronic pain had a mean pain duration of 16.3 years, with 49 per cent of these individuals on medication, and only 9 per cent reported having ever attended a pain clinic. For men reporting pain, no subjects for either age group reported ever having attended a pain clinic. Men in the sixites group indicated a mean duration of chronic pain of 15.8 years with 40 per cent of these individuals reporting that they took medication. The eighties subjects reported chronic pain, with the mean duration being 15.2 years and 50 per cent of those individuals were taking medication for the pain. Factors that might account for the high tolerance

Table 2. The relationship between pain and age

Age group (years)	Pain group	No pain
60–69	40 (30%)	11 (18%)
70–79	70 (47%)	33 (53%)
80–89	28 (21%)	16 (26%)
90 +	5 (2%)	2 (3%)
Total N = 205	N =143	N = 62

of pain by the elderly in this study were, in the first place, a defiant attitude to succumbing to the problems of old age. A second likely factor was almost total absence of psychopathology, specifically clinical depression. There was as well a tendency for this population to deny physical and psychological problems.

The young-old and oldest-old healthy elderly subjects in the above study were compared also on social variables that may influence pain behaviours. Living arrangements were divided into living alone or with spouse and family. There was no significant difference between the two age groups regarding this variable. For the age sixties group, 56 per cent of the subjects reported living alone, and the remainder reported living with a spouse or family. For the age eighties, 69 per cent reported living alone and 31 per cent indicated they lived with a spouse or family. The two elderly groups were compared for activity levels as a social variable in trying to understand differing frequencies of reported pain. Activities were divided into three categories that were not scored as mutually exclusive; (a) social activities, usually organized; (b) visiting family or friends; and (c) physical recreation, such as swimming and dancing. There was a significant difference between groups only for frequency of physical recreational activities. In the sixties group 81 per cent attended social activities, 75 per cent visited regularly with friends and family, and 31 per cent engaged in physical recreational activities. In the eighties group 67 per cent attended social activities, 76 per cent visited regularly with friends and family, but only 2 per cent engaged in physical recreational activities. Finally, health (a self-report of illness within the previous six months requiring at least several days bed rest) was compared. No significant differences between the two elderly groups were found. For the age sixties group, 44 per cent reported recent illness, and 56 per cent did not report illness within the past six months. With the age eighties subjects, 45 per cent reported a recent illness, and 55 per cent indicated no illness.

In summary, the findings from this study (Thomas and Roy, 1988) were that in a sample of 'healthy' elderly the 'oldest-elderly' did not report significantly more pain as a group, compared with a 'younger-elderly' group. Actually, the oldest-elderly reported less chronic pain than the comparison group in their sixties (64 per cent to 81 per cent), while reports of recent illness differed by only 1 per cent between the two age groups. Although the incidence of chronic pain in 'healthy' subjects over sixty-five is about 73 per cent on average, this figure does not support the view, when health status and demographic factors are controlled, that the process of ongoing ageing is associated with increasing disability because of pain. One possible explanation might be that the oldest-old survivors simply enjoy better health than do many of their younger counterparts. However, good physical health is only one, albeit very important, factor. Clearly there is an interaction between denial, clinical depression, and reported pain. It would appear that the older-elderly report less pain, independent of health status, than do the younger-elderly. It seems to be a myth that those individuals who live to be members of the older-elderly group do so at the expense of greater pain and decreasing social interactions.

Age and Pain Relationship

Current research, as the above study has indicated, has found a tentative negative correlation between age and pain. This phenomenon of decreasing pain reports with increasing age is a reversal in the association between age and reported pain found in earlier research that investigated the age and pain relationship.

In earlier research Crook, Rideout, and Brown (1984) in a study on pain in a general population found that report of pain increased with age. The results indicated that 25 per cent of those aged sixty-one to seventy, 29 per cent of those aged seventy-one to eighty, and 40 per cent of those over eighty reported pain. These results were consistent with the general popular perception that increased pain occurred with ageing. A number of large population studies have yielded contradictory results indicating that the elderly in comparison with the young and middle-aged populations report *less* overall pain. Specifically, Harris et al. (1985) found younger individuals report more headache, backache, muscle pain, and stomach and dental pain than the elderly do. Only reports of joint pain increased with advancing age. The *Nuprin Report* (Harris et al., 1985), using a large representative sample from the United States, and Thomas and Roy (1988) and Cook (1992), using Canadian non-stratified samples, both found reports of decreasing pain for headache, neck pain, backache, and muscle, chest, and stomach pain with increasing age. The only exception was increased reports of joint pain with increasing age.

One study that investigated attitudes towards health in the elderly that could help clarify the apparent contradiction between ageing and fewer reported pain experiences was conducted by Prohaska et al. (1985). They surveyed young, middle-aged, and elderly respondents regarding health practices and possible mediating variables that might explain the differences between age cohorts and pain complaints. Prohaska et al. reported that elderly subjects had higher frequencies of engaging in health-promoting actions than younger respondents did. Health-promoting actions consisted of behaviours such as regular medical check-ups, avoidance of salt, regular sleep, and eating a balanced diet. These health behaviours were related to the elderly persons' perceived vulnerability to illness and that illness was felt to be more serious in its possible consequences. Symptoms associated with illness in general by the elderly were tiredness, lack of energy, weakness, and sleeplessness.

Family Relationships and Pain

Another important mediating variable in the formulation of health attitudes, behaviours, and prevalence of pain complaints in the healthy elderly is family relationships. Baranowski and Nader (1985) have shown a positive relationship between family psychological functioning and health-related behaviours. In contrast, findings by Edwards, Zeichner, Kuczmierczyk, and Boczkowski (1985) suggest that the number of pain sufferers (models) in an individual's family and the frequency of pain experiences are also mediating variables for health behaviours. Modelling might account partially for declining pain reports with ageing if, for example, influential role models for the elderly only infrequently give public expression of pain.

Overall, the developmental roots of attitudes towards pain and illness in the healthy elderly remain largely conjectural at this time. The influence of modelling, vicarious conditioning, and personality correlates on pain and illness behaviour have been studied primarily in clinical populations (Gentry, Shows, and Thomas, 1974; Ziesat, 1978; Turkat, 1982; Turkat, Guise, and Carter, 1983; Violon and Giurgen, 1984). The social learning model for predicting influential mediating variables on health attitudes and pain behaviour with both clinical and non-clinical populations has been useful in the literature. This approach allows for explanation of the acquisition of attitudes towards health and pain as well as actual health and pain behaviours.

Thomas et al. (1989), using a social learning model, investigated with a

Table 3. Frequencies of reported pain in the elderly

| | Pain reported once or more | |
	Annually (%)	Weekly (%)
Headache	61	4
Neck	59	3
Back	21	4
Muscle	67	3
Chest	44	1
Stomach	52	1
Joint	85	5
Teeth/ear	28	>1
Nausea	35	1
Cramp	51	2

'healthy' elderly population a number of variables associated with familial and peer modelling as well as personal pain and illness experiences as mediating variables across the life span. In that study the elderly sample (mean age, 71.5 years; range, sixty to eighty-five years; n =124) was composed primarily of the elderly subjects who were ambulatory and living in independent settings (91 per cent). The remaining part of the elderly sample (9 per cent) required home care assistance in their daily activities.

Demographic information (relating to possible pain models) indicated that 49 per cent lived alone and 49 per cent lived with a spouse or family. Additionally, 95 per cent of the elderly reported no living parents with the remaining 5 per cent reporting only one parent alive. Frequencies of social and family interactions for the elderly across a two-week period indicated an average of 5.0 social contacts with family members, 13.6 social contacts with friends, and 26.0 social contacts with acquaintances. The elderly age group had both friends and family members with health problems. The number of family members' pain models was on average 0.90 ($S.D.$ = 1.71). The correlation between number of pain models for the elderly subjects and reported frequencies for ten different locations for pain was significant. Specifically, there were significant correlations between the number of reported heart problem models and perceived vulnerability to heart attack as well as cancer models and perceived vulnerability to cancer. Especially strong was the correlation between number of family models and degree of expressed worry about developing arthritis in the elderly. Table 3 shows the frequencies of reported pain in the elderly group.

This particular finding that the numbers of familial and peer pain models (with specific illness) were related to perceptions of vulnerability and worries regarding these same illnesses suggests one of the origins of attitudes regarding health for the elderly. A second finding in this study was that the number of familial pain models was positively correlated with the frequency of pain complaints. The possibility of denial with the so-called healthy elderly is likely, because the literature reports that the elderly in general tend to experience pain as a part of everyday life (Roy and Thomas, 1986). In conclusion, the impact of opportunities to witness the responses of peers and family to illness and pain can be substantial and lasting (Craig, 1978).

CONCLUSION

First, it is important to keep in perspective the proper context surrounding the relationship between pain and health in the age group defined as elderly. The basic relationship between physical dysfunction as the cause of pain is the same for the elderly population as it is for all other age groups. Pain in the elderly is caused by specific disease and/or chronic illness conditions. There is no empirical evidence of a direct or an indirect link between physical causes for pain and age, independent of health status. However, there are distinctive differences in health behaviours such as frequency and locations of reported pain that are consistently associated with different age groups of healthy individuals.

The differences in reported pain experiences between the healthy elderly and healthy individuals in other age groups is generally assumed to be variable because of social and psychological factors. The trend is that with ageing, a person generally becomes more conscious of health issues, this transition in attitudes and behaviour becomes notable for most North Americans as they progress through their forties, when it is common for most individuals (healthy as well as ill) to become aware of structural and functional changes occurring in relation to the process of the biological ageing of the human body.

Accompanying the increasing attention to health with ageing is a decreasing reporting of pain. This phenomenon among healthy individuals becomes so notable that comparisons between young and elderly age groups find statistically significant differences in frequency, duration, and number of locations with pain complaints. Considering the findings of Leventhal and Prohaska (1986) age-related differences in reported pain are not surprising. Leventhal and Prohaska found that the elderly develop attitudes, not present (as strongly) at younger ages, that pain and illness represent serious threats to health. Psychological defense mechanisms such as denial may, in part, account for such findings. However, work by Roy and Thomas (1986, 1987, 1988) in a group of studies investigating pain in the elderly did not find that denial alone accounted for lower frequencies in reported pain in a healthy elderly population. Thomas and Roy (1988) further found that decreased reports of pain with increasing age occurred within the elderly group as well, going from the youngest-old to the oldest-old. Variables such as stimulus habituation, differential social reinforcement, and depression are unable to explain age differences in pain reporting between healthy elderly individuals and other age groups. It would appear at this time that the explanation for decreased reporting of pain with increasing age is a complex phenomenon likely involving psychological, social, and probably biological variables.

Many diseases are age specific in prevalence rates of onset. For example, children have the highest rates of chicken pox and measles, teenagers and young adults have the highest rates for schizophrenia and headaches, middle-aged individuals have the highest rates of back pain and cancer, while the elderly have the highest rates of arthritis and neurological disorders. Thus, differences in reported pain between younger-old and oldest-old healthy elderly are not totally surprising. Also, illness whether temporary or chronic is not synonymous with pain.

It is important to remember that there is more variation in physical health status among the elderly than for any other age group, thus making valid generalizations about the healthy elderly difficult. Additional confounding issues include possible side-effect interactions between multiple medications frequently prescribed to the elderly, biased beliefs and attitudes about pain and health in the elderly, and lack of uniformity in definitions and procedures in the research literature on pain in the elderly. There is an empirically demonstrated positive association between health risk factors and ageing based on measures of prevalence of serious diseases in the research literature. It is not established whether (a) consistent relationships exist between shifts in physical sensory threshold with ageing; (b) increased general versus specific pain experiences occur as a function of ageing; and (c) increasing psychological dysfunction as a result of ageing biases pain reporting. These and many other factors help determine baseline expectations for the healthy elderly when trying to identify and describe this population.

An individual of any age who is described as 'healthy' is typically viewed as pain free. However, as the literature reviewed in this chapter has shown, this is a misperception with the elderly. Frequent pain appears to be present in individuals at all ages including the elderly. The perception is that an elderly individual who is 'healthy' is relatively independent of pain except in the most chronic and severe instances of pain experiences. Pain in clinical populations as well as in the 'healthy' elderly is currently conceptualized as being multidimensional: physical, psychological, and social. In the healthy elderly sensory thresholds are not currently seen as responsible for the variance between reports of pain and measures of physical neurological stimuli that communicate pain. Changes in memory, intelligence, and psychological functioning when health status is controlled for do not explain frequency and intensity variations in reports of pain in the healthy elderly. Clinical pain populations, especially the young and middle-aged chronic pain suffers, as well as the healthy elderly are likely all to benefit greatly if the coping process can be understood that results in less reported and possibly less perceived pain as individuals age and reach the elderly life stage.

REFERENCES

Baranowski, T., & Nader, P. (1985). Family health behavior. In: D. Turk & R.D. Kerns (eds.), *Health, Illness, and Families: A Life-Span, Perspective*, New York: Wiley, 51–80.

Brody, E., Kleban, M., & Moles, E. (1983). What older people do about their day-to-day mental and physical health symptoms. *Journal of the American Geriatric Society, 31*, 89–98.

Buskist, W., & Gerbing, D.W. (1990). *Psychology: Boundaries and Frontiers.* Glenview, Il: Scott, Foresman / Little, Brown Higher Education.

Craig, K.D. (1978). Social modelling influences on pain. In: R.A. Sternbach (Ed.), *The Psychology of Pain.* New York: Raven Press.

Crook, J., Rideout, E., & Browne, G. (1984). The prevalence of pain complaints in a general population. *Pain, 18*, 299–314.

Cutler, S.J., & Grams, A.E. (1988). Correlates of self-reported everyday memory complaints. *Journal of Gerontology, 43*, 582–90.

Demlow, L., Laing, M., & Eaton, H. (1986). Impact of chronic arthritis on the elderly. *Clinical Rheumatic Disorders, 12*, 329.

Edwards, P., Zeichner, A., Kuczmierczyk, A., & Boczkowski, J. (1985). Familial pain models: The relationship between family history of pain and current pain experience. *Pain, 21*, 379–84.

Ferrell, B.A. (1991). Pain management in elderly people. *American Geriatric Society, 39*, 64–73.

Fry, P.S., & Wong, P.T.P. (1991). Pain management training in the elderly: Matching interventions with subjects' coping styles. *Stress Medicine, 7*, 93–8.

Gentry, W., Shows, W.D., & Thomas, M.R. (1974). Chronic low back pain: A psychological profile. *Psychosomatics, 15*, 174–7.

Gilewski, M.J., & Zelinski, E.M. (1986). Questionnaire assessment of memory complaints. In: L.W. Poon (Ed.), *Handbook for Clinical Memory Assessment of Older Adults.* Washington DC: American Psychological Association.

Gochman, D.S. (1985). Family determinants of children's concepts of health and illness. In: D. Turk, & R.D. Kerns (Eds.), *Health, Illness, and Families: A Life-Span Perspective.* New York: Wiley, 1–22.

Guralnik, J.M., Yanagashita, M., & Schneider, E.I. (1988). Projecting the older population of the United States: Lessons from the past and prospects for the future. *Millbank Quarterly, 66*, 283–308.

Haley, W.E., & Dolce, J.J. (1986). Assessment and management of chronic pain in the elderly. *Clinical Gerontology 5*, 435–55.

Harkins, S.W. (1988). Pain in the elderly. In: R. Dubner, G.F. Gebhart, & M.R. Bond (Eds.), *Pain Research and Clinical Management*, vol. 3. Amsterdam: Elsevier.

Harris, D.M., & Guten, S. (1979). Health protective behavior: An exploratory study. *Journal of Health and Social Behaviour, 20*, 17–29.

Harris, L., & Associates (1985). *The Nuprin Pain Report.* New York: Louis Harris and Associates.

Hulicka, I.M. (1967). Short-term learning and memory efficiency as a function of age and health. *Journal of the American Geriatric Society, 15*, 285–94.

Kaplan, G., Barell, V., & Lusky, A. (1988). Subjective state of health and survival in elderly adults. *Journal of Gerontology: Social Sciences, 43*, 114–20.

Keefe, F.J., & Williams, D.A. (1990). A comparison of coping strategies in chronic pain patients in different age groups. *Journal of Gerontology: Psychological Sciences, 45*, 161–5.

Lau, R.R. (1982). Origins of health locus of control beliefs. *Journal Personal and Social Psychology, 42*, 322–34.

Leventhal, E., & Prohaska, T.R. (1986). Age, symptom interpretation, and health behavior. *Journal of the American Geriatrics Society, 34*, 185–91.

Melding, P.S. (1991). Is there such a thing as geriatric pain? *Pain, 46*, 119–21.

Parmelee, P.A., Katz, I.R., & Lawton, M.P. (1989). Depression among institutionalized aged: Assessment and prevalence estimation. *Journal of Gerontology: Medical Sciences, 44*, 22–9.

Parmelee, P.A., Katz, I.R., & Lawton, M.P. (1991). The relation of pain to depression among institutionalized aged. *Journal of Gerontology: Psychological Sciences, 46*, 15–21.

Peterson, C., & Seligman, M.E.P. (1984). Causal explanations as a risk factor for depression: Theory and evidence. *Psychological Review, 91*, 347–74.

Poon, L.W. (1985). Differences in human memory with aging: Nature, causes, and clinical implications. In: J.E. Birren & K.W. Schaie (Eds.), *Handbook of the Psychology of Aging*. New York: Van Nostrand-Reinhold.

Prohaska, T., Keller, M., Leventhal, E., and Leventhal, H. (1987). Impact of symptoms and aging attribution on emotions and coping. *Health Psychology, 6*, 495–514.

Prohaska, T., Laventhal, E., Laventhal, H., & Keller, M. (1985). Health practices and illness cognition in young middle-aged and elderly adults. *Journal of Gerontology, 40*, 569–78.

Roy, R., & Thomas, M.R. (1986). A survey of chronic pain in an elderly population. *Canadian Family Physicians, 31*, 513–16.

Roy, R., & Thomas, M. (1987). Elderly persons with and without pain: A comparative study (Part I). *Clinical Journal of Pain, 3*, 102–6.

Roy, R., & Thomas, M. (1988). Pain, depression, and illness behavior in a group of community based elderly persons: Elderly persons with and without pain (Part II). *Clinical Journal of Pain, 3*, 207–11.

Roy, R., & Thomas, M. (1989). Memories of pain: Comparison of 'worst pain ever' experienced by senior citizens and college students. *Clinical Journal of Pain, 5*, 359–62.

Roy, R., Thomas, M., & Berger, S. (1990). A comparative study of Canadian nonclinical and British pain clinic subjects. *Clinical Jouirnal of Pain, 6*, 276–83.

Roy, R., Thomas, M., & Makarenko, P. (1990). A comparative study of pain complaints in a non-clinical Canadian population of university students and seniors. *Pain Clinics, 3*, 213–22.

Roy, R., Thomas, M., & Matas, M. (1984). Chronic pain and clinical depression: A review. *Comprehensive Psychiatry, 25*, 96–105.

Schaie, K.W. (1982). Longitudinal methods. In B.B. Wolman (Ed.), *Handbook of Developmental Psychology*. Englewood Cliffs, NJ: Prentice-Hall.

Schaie, K.W., & Willis, S.L. (1986). *Adult Development and Aging*. Boston: Little Brown.

Sunderland, A., Watts, K., Baddeley, A.D., & Harris, J.E. (1986). Subjective memory assessment and test performance in elderly adults. *Journal of Gerontology, 41*, 376–84.

Thomas, M., & Roy, R. (1988). Age and pain: A comparative study of younger versus older elderly persons. *Journal of Pain Management Practice, 4*, 174–9.

Thomas, M.R., Roy, R., & Cook, A. (1992). Reports of family pain by college students including a subsample of pain reports of parents. *Pain Clinics, 5*, 137–45.

Thomas, M., Roy, R., & Makarenko, P. (1989). Social modelling in attitudes toward pain and illness: A comparison of young and elderly subjects. *Journal of Pain Management, 2*, 309–15.

Tucker, M.A., Andrew, M.F., Ogle, S.J., & Davison, J.G. (1989). Age-associated change in pain threshold measured by transcutaneous neuronal electrical stimulation. *Age and Aging, 18*, 241–6.

Turkat, I.D. (1982). An investigation of parental modelling in the etiology of diabetic illness behavior. *Behavior Research and Therapy, 20*, 547–52.

Turkat, I.D., Guise, B.J., & Carter, K.M. (1983). The effects of vicarious experience on pain termination and work avoidance: A replication. *Behavior Research and Therapy, 21*, 491–3.

United States Bureau of the Census (1986). *Statistical Brief.* Washington, DC: United States Government Printing Office.

Violon, A., & Giurgen, D. (1984). Familial models for chronic pain. *Pain, 18*, 199–203.

Waddell, G. (1987). A new clinical model for the treatment of low-back pain. *Spine, 12*, 632–44.

Ziesat, H.A. (1978). Are family patterns related to the development of chronic low backpain? *Perception of Motor Skills, 46*, 1062.

4

Pain Management in the Elderly

BRUCE A. SORKIN and DENNIS C. TURK

There is no doubt that pain is a problem that pervades all age groups including the elderly. Studies in settings as diverse as Canada (Crook, Rideout, and Browne, 1984), the United States (Hale, Perkins, May, Marks, and Stewart, 1986), Europe (Brattberg, Mats, and Anders, 1989; Österlind, Lofgren, Sandman, Steen, and Winblad, 1986), and Asia (Lau-Ting and Phoon, 1988) all attest to the fact that pain is common and debilitating to the elderly. The consequences of pain in the elderly include depression, decreased socialization, sleep disturbance, impaired ambulation and increased health care costs, deconditioning, falls, slow rehabilitation, polypharmacy, cognitive dysfunction, and malnutrition (Ferrell, 1991). Yet, surprisingly little research has been devoted specifically to the problem of geriatric pain and its management. Ferrell notes that of the eleven leading textbooks of geriatric medicine, only two include chapters on pain management. He further notes that a review of eight geriatric nursing texts reveals that fewer than eighteen of five thousand pages (0.36 per cent) were devoted to the treatment of pain.

Geriatric patients are underserved at all points in the treatment process. Harkins and Price (1993) cite that fewer than 8 per cent of 174 patients evaluated at a pain centre were over sixty-five years of age, whereas the percentage of people above sixty-five in the general population is 13. One may well question why such discrepancies exist. Some pain centres set an upper limit on the age of patients they will accept, citing either a preconceived notion that pain management is inappropriate for elderly patients *per se* because of physical or cognitive limitations or that the elderly pain patient is not employed and that a major purpose of the program is to facilitate the return to work.

Another reason for the lack of attention to the geriatric pain patient is that where data are lacking, 'myth' will fill the vacuum. In many cases our personal and professional mythologies or stereotypes are helpful, because they are based on reasonable extrapolations from data and have considerable heuristic value. But there are cases in which our assumptions and the 'conventional wisdom' are wrong, and, worse, these assumptions are not benign. Geriatric patients have been portrayed as docile, regressed, and rigid in their approach to problem solving. For example, Pfeiffer (1977) in the *Handbook of the Psychology of Aging*, says that older people often revert to a 'more primitive style of coping' marked by unmodified anxiety, depression–withdrawal, projection, somatization, and denial. Gutmann (1970) describes older men as passing through a sequence of coping from active to passive to 'magical mastery,' in which coping is described as being tantamount to 'hoping that it's all a bad dream.' Older people have been characterized by practitioners as early as Freud as being 'anti-introspective' and lacking the personal qualities necessary for psychological intervention or the interest in pursuing it.

Gatz and Pearson (1988) described elderly patients as being 'stuck between a rock and a hard place' when it comes to pain. An elderly patient complaining of pain may not be referred for specialty treatment, because the primary care physician sees pain as a normal aspect of ageing not amenable to treatment. In fact, Ferrell (1991) cites the importance of adequately questioning elderly patients about pain, because even patients themselves may fail to report it because they ascribe their symptoms to the natural process of ageing and 'don't want to bother' the doctor. Additionally, pain may have existed for such a long period that older adults may not be able to recall a time when symptoms were absent. In this case, they may be unable to identify their present symptoms as abnormal or atypical.

Even when pain *is* recognized, however, as being pathological, patients who otherwise might be referred to a multidisciplinary centre for pain may be referred only for medication management, because they are assumed to be suffering from Alzheimer's disease or some other cognitive impairment or physical limitation that makes them poor candidates for rehabilitation. This possibility seems especially likely because of the high co-morbidity between pain and depression in the elderly (Lipton, Pfeffer, Newman, and Soloman, 1993; Williamson and Schulz, 1992) and given that pain itself might compromise cognitive performance (Ferrell, 1991; Harkins and Price, 1993).

Sorkin (1993) reported data that contradict assertions about pain and decline in cognitive performance being specific to elderly versus younger pain patients. An index of cognitive impairment was created using three items drawn from the SCL90-R (Derogatis, 1992). These items assessed memory, cognitive blocking, and concentration difficulty with the items 'Trouble remembering things,' 'Your mind going blank,' and 'Trouble concentrating,' respectively. A group of elderly patients ($n = 5$; mean age = 63.8 years) and younger patients ($n = 9$; mean age = 24.2) patients had comparable scores on this index. Although differences did not even approach significance, ($t[12] = - .60$; $p = .56$), the trends in the data were for the *younger* patients to report more problems with cognitive clarity. Scores on the Cognitive Impairment Index could range from zero (no problems) to 12 (extreme problems in all areas of cognitive function). The mean of the elderly group was 3.6 ($SD = 1.3$), whereas the mean for the younger group was 4.6 ($SD = 3.4$). Furthermore, when examined by means of a regression analysis using twenty-eight subjects ranging in age from twenty to seventy-two, there was no significant correlation between age and total scores on the Cognitive Impairment Index ($r_{28} = - .12$; $p < .53$) or for the question about memory alone ($r_{28} = .07$; $p < .74$).

Differences clearly were present when the pain patients as a whole were compared with population norms as reported in the *SCL-90-R Administration, Scoring and Procedures Manual-II* (Derogatis, 1992). Chi-square analyses indicated that pain patients more frequently complained of concentration problems and mental blocking. Differences on the item inquiring about memory problems reached only the .053 level of probability, although the trend was for patients in pain to acknowledge greater difficulty with memory.

The results of the Sorkin (1993) study support the contention that chronic pain is associated with increased reports of cognitive impairments. Patients with pain more frequently reported that they had difficulties with concentration and blocking. There was a strong trend towards reporting more frequent and severe memory problems. As suggested by other authors, this could lead to increased perceptions of cognitive frailty and to false positive identification of dementia. Nevertheless, the present data suggest that both older and younger patients are affected equally. It seems most parsimonious to conclude that many of these deficits are caused by the distraction associated with pain or by other confounding factors such as sleep deprivation, use of medication, fatigue, feelings of helplessness, or affective disorder. The important implication from this is that, as in the case of pseudodementia associated with depression, the cognitive impairments seen may diminish as the pain is decreased or as complicating factors (such as polypharmacy) are eliminated.

The results of the Sorkin study (1993) suggest that it is important to examine some of the many assumptions made about the ageing pain population. We hope to further address this and some of the other perceptions of the geriatric patient with pain in the present chapter. Specifically, are there differences in the outcomes of pain management for older and younger patients? Do older patients have a different and inherently inferior approach to solving problems in their lives that makes them unable to benefit from treatment? Finally, should we modify the treatment of older pain patients in order to improve outcomes?

DO OLDER AND YOUNGER PATIENTS DIFFER IN THEIR
TYPICAL WAYS OF DEALING WITH STRESS?

There are two types of theories that predict differences in the ways that older and younger people confront stress. These are referred to as developmental and contextual theories (Folkman, Lazarus, Pimley, and Novacek, 1987).

Contextual Theory

The contextual theory portrays differences in coping, when they do occur, as being the result of the different stresses faced by ageing individuals. Differences in coping therefore are not the result of biological changes but rather they are an artefact of the various environmental pressures placed on individuals over the life span. In terms of the 'nature–nurture' dichotomy, this would be cast on the 'nurture' pole. The stresses experienced by older and younger individuals change across the life span. Older people deal with more 'exit' events such as death and retirement, compared with 'entrance' events such as marriage, birth, and new jobs, which are commonly experienced by younger people.

Stresses of different types may be more appropriately dealt with through different strategies. Stress that is essentially unchangeable is best dealt with through modification of the way one feels about it. For example, if a person is short and feels self-conscious about it, he or she cannot grow by exerting sheer force of will but instead must deal with the stress by changing the way he or she feels about being short. Similar remarks can be made for dealing with the fact that one's spouse has been diagnosed with Alzheimer's disease or colon cancer. Other situations are more changeable. If one has a leaking roof, the effective strategy is to fix it and not merely to grow to love being wet.

Developmental Theories

Developmental theories suggest that differences are an inherent part of the normal process of ageing. Similar to the cognitive changes described by Piaget or the changes in moral thought described by Kulberg or Gilligan, different developmental stages are associated with different characteristic coping patterns. We can portray this position as the 'nature' hypothesis, because it suggests that there is some quasibiological process underlying the changes and, furthermore, that the changes should be evident across a variety of social and cultural contexts.

There are three positions within the developmental interpretation, each of which makes specific and mutually exclusive predictions about coping. The regression position holds that people become more primitive in their coping styles as they grow older. They become more self-absorbed, impulsive, hostile, and show less ability to tolerate anxiety. The opposite view, the growth position, holds that people become more mature as they age, and they will normally show greater ego strength as exemplified by utilizing conscious suppression, humour, wisdom, and caring for others. A third perspective based on Jungian theory suggests that men and women will show divergent tendencies as they age, with men becoming more passive and less aggressive with age and women becoming more active and aggressive (Folkman et al., 1987).

DIFFERENTIAL RESPONSES TO LIFE STRESSES BY AGE

Folkman et al. (1987) examined the types of major life stresses and common daily problems experienced by older (mean age, sixty-eight) and younger (mean age, forty) subjects and the ways they dealt with them. Subjects tracked the stress they encountered and described their coping behaviours using the Ways of Coping Scale (Folkman and Lazarus, 1985). This scale contains a wide array of cognitive and behavioural coping strategies. Subjects were asked to rate the degree to which they employed each strategy when they were dealing with a recent difficulty. Examples of items from the Ways of Coping Scale can be seen in Table 1.

There were definite differences between the two age cohorts on both the number of problems faced and the proportion of problems each problem group represented. For example, the older group had a smaller absolute number of problems associated with home maintenance, but given that they also had an overall lower rate of problems, the proportion of total problems accounted for by home maintenance was actually higher. Regard-

Table 1. Examples of items from the Ways of Coping Scale (Folkman & Lazarus, 1985)

Strategy	Example
Confrontive coping	Stood my ground and fought for what I wanted.
Self-control	I tried to keep my feelings to myself.
Distancing	Went on as if nothing had happened.
Seek social support	Talked to someone who could do something concrete about the problem.
Accept responsibility	Realized I brought the problem on myself.
Escape/avoidance	Wished that the situation would go away or somehow be over with.
Planful problem solving	I made a plan of action and followed it.
Positive reappraisal	Found new faith.

ing the number of life events and difficulties faced by both groups, the younger group reported more problems having to do with finances, work, home maintenance, personal life, and family and friends. As a proportion of the total problems, the younger group reported relatively more difficulties with finance. Younger subjects reported that work accounted for a larger percentage of their problems (which was only to be expected given that subjects in the older group were almost always retired). The older group reported a higher proportion of problems having to do with environmental and social pressures as well as home maintenance. The older group had more health problems.

With respect to the ways of coping with stress, the younger group reported using more confrontational coping and sought more social support. They used less distancing and positive reappraisal. Looking at ways of coping for specific problem domains, in most areas, older subjects tended to use more distancing, more positive reappraisal, accepted more responsibility, and used less confrontational coping or planful problem solving. However, in the matter of health concerns, older people were more confrontational than younger people, and there was no difference in the use of escape–avoidance for this source of stress.

The observed differences in coping failed to clearly support either a growth or regression developmental position but instead seemed to be a blend of coping skills. The only position to receive no support was the Jungian theory. There was no evidence to suggest divergent styles in older men and women. It was difficult to assess the precise differences in the ways the two samples dealt with health matters, because as defined in the Folkman et al. study (1987), health problems ranged from problems with weight to terminal cancer. Several other studies, however, have specifically addressed ways that older patients cope with illness and pain.

McCrae (1982) examined coping and stresses in 423 men and 129 women involved in the Baltimore Longitudinal Study of Aging. Also included were 183 wives and 16 husbands of these people. Subjects in the Baltimore study were highly educated with 25 per cent holding doctorates and 71 per cent holding college degrees. Thus, we need to exercise some caution in generalizing beyond this sample. Subjects in Study 1 (McCrae, 1982) had been regularly contacted for medical and psychological testing since 1958.

Subjects completed a checklist of life events covering the preceding year. Life events were classified as losses, threats, or challenges. Events were ranked for stressfulness using the Social Readjustment Rating Scale (Holmes and Rahe, 1967). Subjects were assigned to different groups (threat, loss, or challenge) randomly, unless only one type of event had occurred to them. Subjects were asked to recall the assigned stressor. They then read a series of 118 items describing ways of coping with stress and were asked to indicate which of them they had employed during the course of the stressor. The 118 items were grouped by factor analysis into twenty-eight coping mechanisms.

Analyses of variance using three age groups (young, twenty-four to forty-nine; middle, fifty to sixty-four; and elderly, sixty-five to ninety-one) revealed that for these twenty-eight coping mechanisms, there were only ten significant ($p < .05$) differences. Contrary to predictions made by the regression position, older patients were not different from younger patients in their use of isolation of affect, intellectual denial, wishful thinking, or passivity, and they were actually *lower* regarding the use of self-blame, withdrawal, and assessing blame. Although the decreases in self-blame, withdrawal, and assessing blame were consistent with the growth position, none of the 'mature' mechanisms such as substitution, restraint, or rational action showed the increases with age consistent with the growth position and one mechanism, humour, decreased with age.

Challenges decreased significantly with age. Losses occurred at all ages with equal frequency. Threats, however, increased with age. Differences (or lack thereof), therefore, may be the result of the different stresses encountered by the groups. When the nature of the stress was controlled for, there were decreases in hostile reaction, escapist fantasy, sedation, assessing blame, wishful thinking, and indecisiveness. Increases in the use of faith were also noted.

In a second study (McCrae, 1982) subjects were asked to imagine themselves in three hypothetical situations contrived by the experimenters involving loss, challenge, and threat. The results indicated that older individuals employed declines in hostile reaction, positive thinking, escapist fantasy, restraint, self-adaptation, and humour.

Across both of the McCrae (1982) studies the most consistent declines were in the use of aggression and escapist fantasy. More than half of the twenty-eight mechanisms measured in these studies showed no evidence of age differences. McCrae summarized these results saying: 'A prevalent stereotype about aging individuals is that they lack the ability to adapt to stressful situations. Older individuals are often portrayed as being rigid in their responses or as using regressive defense mechanisms that distort reality instead of dealing effectively with it. The data from these two studies provide no support for this contention. In most respects older people in these studies cope in much the same way as younger people' (p. 459).

Studies Specifically Examining Coping with Pain and Illness

Downe-Wamboldt (1991) studied coping skills in a group of ninety community-residing Canadian women aged sixty-five or greater, diagnosed with osteoarthritis (OA). The women in her study reported using a variety of strategies including emotive, palliative, and confrontational. Women who relied on emotive coping strategies, however, tended to have lower scores on ratings of life satisfaction. It is clear that the women studied engaged in a variety of coping strategies. However, it is difficult to assess differences in coping between age groups given that a younger cohort was not studied.

Davis, Cortez, and Rubin (1990) examined the use of coping skills in older (mean age, seventy-two) and younger (mean age, forty-nine) patients with OA or rheumatoid arthritis (RA). They reported that older patients and younger patients seemed to have a similar size coping repertoire with the older patients mentioning an average of seven coping skills, whereas the younger patients averaged nine. Both groups relied primarily on physically based methods of pain relief including rest, massage, heat, and medication. The younger group rated relaxation as being of significantly greater benefit. A significant confound in the study was that the younger group was over-represented by patients with RA versus OA, and it is difficult to know whether or not differences in coping were the result of diagnosis or age.

In a study by Sorkin, Rudy, Hanlon, Turk, and Stieg (1990), older patients and younger patients were interviewed during an initial assessment at a pain treatment facility. Older patients did not differ from younger patients in terms of the number of enumerated physically based coping strategies. There was a statistically significant, albeit small tendency for the older patients to name fewer cognitive coping strategies (older mean = .46; younger mean = .96). Neither group named many cognitive skills, and this supports the findings reported by Davis et al. (1990) who used a recognition strategy (asking patients to identify how often they used a specified technique) versus the recall strategy used in the Sorkin et at. (1990) study (asking how patients cope using an open-ended format).

A study by Fry and Wong (1991) examined the ability of training in coping skills to affect pain levels in subjects aged sixty-three to eighty-two. Subjects were assigned to problem-focused or emotion-focused training according to their pre-existing coping styles. They also examined whether subjects who preferred and received training in problem-focused coping performed more effectively than persons preferring and receiving emotion-based problem-solving skills. Although Fry and Wong (1991) did not report the results of individual comparisons, visual inspection of their data suggests that patients in the emotion-focused group had the best initial results in terms of pain reduction, anxiety, satisfaction, and adjustment. However, patients in the problem-focused group appeared to be doing the best after a two-month follow-up. These results suggest that geriatric patients who prefer coping styles that centre on control of their emotional reactions do best when they are in active treatment and are probably receiving a good deal of reinforcement and support from the treatment team. When there is a hiatus in this support, they appear to backslide, whereas the problem-focused group continues to improve. It remains an empirical question, however, as to whether emotion-focused patients would improve with an intervention consisting of problem-focused strategies and whether they too would have shown a trend towards continuing improvement. It should be noted that subjects in the Fry and Wong study (1991) were not randomly assigned to interventions and that this is a serious flaw that limits the interpretation of the results. Another serious problem in the study was failure to assess the actual frequency with which the different groups used the proffered skills. One cannot be certain that subjects exposed to training in emotion-focused skills either learned or performed the skills above their baseline level.

Felton and Revenson (1987) interviewed adults over the age of forty who had one of four serious illnesses including hypertension, diabetes, RA, or one of three systemic blood cancers. The subjects also were interviewed over the telephone using a subset of questions approximately seven months after the initial interview. Coping measures were derived through a factor analysis of the Ways of Coping Scale (Folkman and Lazarus, 1985). The six scales included information seeking, cognitive restructuring, emotional expression, wish-fulfilling fantasy, threat minimization, and self-blame. Felton and Revenson concluded that age plays a role in determining the choice of a coping strategy, although its influence is limited in scope and modest in strength. As in the Folkman et al. (1987) and the McCrae (1982) studies, older adults were less likely to use emotional expression as a coping technique. They were also less likely to engage in information seeking than were middle-aged adults in their efforts to cope with illness.

Felton and Revenson (1987) and Folkman et al. were not alone in noting that elderly persons tend to engage in less information seeking and to demand less control in problem-solving situations. Haug (1979), Cassileth, Zupkis, Sutton-Smith, and March (1980), and Woodward and Wallston (1987) all reported that older patients have lower desires for control over their health care decisions.

Woodward and Wallston (1987) suggest that either cohort effects or developmental changes (such as cognitive decline) or both could account for the change in desire for control. Also of potential importance is self-efficacy. Older people may desire less control, because they feel less able to effectively manage the information. Woodward and Wallston reported that older subjects had lower ratings of self-efficacy for managing health-related decisions. Elderly subjects also expressed less confidence in their ability to handle day-to-day matters as well. This decreased efficacy can lead elderly patients to withdraw from efforts to manage their symptoms.

Summary and Conclusions

When considering the issue of stress and coping, it is helpful to think of both the *mechanisms* of coping, such as constructive actions of escapist fantasies, as well as the *nature* of the stresses confronted. Older and younger people have different lifestyles and face different stresses. Older people encounter more exit events in their lives caused by deaths of family members and friends. Older individuals are not working and do not have the network of peers found at the work-place. They have more frequent illnesses and more frequently require medication for these illnesses. Older individuals often have lower incomes than younger individuals.

The majority of the studies reviewed suggest that older and younger people are substantially similar in their use of coping strategies to deal with stress. In the McCrae study, only ten of twenty-eight strategies were used differentially. The Davis et al. study (1990) indicated that both older and younger persons relied on physical methods to manage pain. This was replicated using a different methodological approach in the Sorkin et al. study (1990). Nevertheless, some differences do reliably occur. Older individuals are less aggressive, use less escapist fantasy, solicit less information about their care, and in general demand less control over their medical care. Woodward and Wallston (1987) suggest that older persons feel less capable of making good decisions about their care and therefore have a greater desire for decisions to be made for them by competent others. It is difficult to know if their perceptions of lower ability are accurate or if they systematically underestimate their skills, because no study has investigated this decision-making ability.

Two studies reported that older individuals who rely on emotion-focused strategies for stress management had less favourable outcomes (Downe-Wamboldt, 1991; Fry and Wong, 1991). There is, however, an interesting 'Catch-22' regarding this result. One form of emotional expression is acknowledging and communicating about one's symptoms and disability. Subjects who prefer emotional expression may simply then be predisposed to acknowledge problems. Optimally, one would want to verify patients' perceptions of their functioning using an independent source. But assuming that their report is accurate, the poorer outcome of this group might be attributed not to the fact that emotional expression is innately inferior, but to the fact that older people generally have fewer social supports. This especially holds true for older individuals who have moved from their neighbourhoods to a residential care facility or for those who have lost a spouse, sibling, or friend, retired recently, or begun to isolate themselves because of problems associated with hearing or visual loss. An interesting question is whether older people who prefer or who use a predominantly emotion-based strategy would do well if maintained within a formal or informal support network.

ARE THERE SPECIFIC ISSUES IN GERIATRIC ASSESSMENT?

As we noted in the previous section on stress and coping, older patients and younger patients share more similarities than differences. For example, both older and younger subjects find that if their pain impairs their ability to perform their usual roles, they experience increased depression. Although this basic process holds for both groups, there are noted differences *in the life experiences typical of older and younger individuals*. These differences are essential to look at because they become part of the social nexus within which the patient's pain exists.

During the multidisciplinary evaluation of the geriatric pain patient, numerous physical abnormalities will likely be noted. It is essential to avoid over-interpreting these findings. For example, Swezey (1988) notes that geriatric patients often can present with symptoms of sciatica and have a positive x-ray of the lower back showing spinal stenosis. However, this is not necessarily indicative of the need for surgery. He claims that the results of conservative treatment in a series of thirty patients with spinal stenosis, eleven of whom had associated acute to subacute sciatic radiculopathy, were 'amazingly good.' Ten of eleven patients recovered and only one needed surgical intervention. In the Sorkin et al. study (1990), older patients presented with larger numbers of physical abnormalities, yet they did not show higher levels of pain or pain-related life impairments. This again indicates the necessity of assessing multiple aspects of the patient's pain experience.

The report of pain is not solely the result of biomedical factors (Turk and Rudy, 1987). Melzack (1975) aptly analogized the process of evaluating pain by stating, 'To describe pain solely in terms of intensity is like specifying the visual world only in terms of light flux without regard to pattern, colour, texture, and the many other dimensions of the visual experience' (p. 278). Pain not only involves an intensity dimension, but also emotional and motivational aspects. When patients in our clinic are asked what their goals are, most respond, 'To get rid of my pain and get my life back to normal.' Through this answer, the patients are acknowledging the importance of the impact of pain on their lifestyles. Patients recognize that pain has adversely affected their mood, hobbies, work habits, sleep, social relationships, spiritual practices and beliefs, sexual activities, and so forth. These aspects therefore are essential to examine when assessing the geriatric pain patient. When evaluating the geriatric patient, there will not necessarily be different methods or content areas, but the nature of the responses one receives may well be different by virtue of the different stresses as well as life experiences encountered by geriatric patients.

Melzack's description (1975) aside, it is essential to make some quantitative assessment of the amount of discomfort experienced by the patient. This can best be done using a pain intensity scale such as that found in the McGill Pain Questionnaire (MPQ; Melzack, 1975) or the Multidimensional Pain Inventory (MPI; Kerns, Turk, and Rudy, 1985). At the very least one should repeatedly measure present pain intensity on a visual analogue scale (Jensen and Karoly, 1992). Pain is an inherently subjective phenomenon, and the best way to assess the presence of pain is to simply ask the patient. One should also feel comfortable accepting the geriatric patient's assessment of the level of discomfort without worrying that the rating has been distorted in some systematic way by a geriatric versus younger pain threshold difference. Harkins and Price (1992), Harkins, Price, and Martelli (1986), and Harkins, Kwentus, and Price (1984) essentially dismiss the existence of clinically significant differences in pain threshold.

A fuller picture of the effect of pain on the patient's life can be gathered by careful interviewing of the patient. We have found it to be especially useful to include a significant other of the geriatric patient in this interview process. Interview data are often gathered through unstructured interviews. We have found, however, that more reliable data are obtained by using a semistructured interview format (Sorkin, Gavlak, Hanlon, and Feldman, 1993 or see Fishbain, Cutler, Rosomoff, and Rosomoff, 1994, for an alternative). The primary areas of inquiry from this interview are presented in Table 2.[1]

The MPQ (Melzack, 1975) further adds to the clinician's understanding of the patient's pain by providing information relevant to the affective and motivational components of pain. The MPI (Kerns et al., 1985) can be quite helpful because it provides a quantitative assessment of factors including the interference in daily activities associated with pain, patients' perceptions of their ability to control important aspects of their lives, patients' rating of their daily activity levels, and their experienced level of emotional distress. The MPI also provides an assessment of the level of social support experienced by patients as well as their perceptions of the degree to which significant others react with hostility or helpfulness and how often they distract the patient from discomfort. Although specific age norms are not available for either of these instruments, data from the Sorkin et al. paper (1990) as well as from the original Kerns et al. description of the MPI suggest that age differences do not occur.

Given the high incidence of depression in the geriatric patient population (Williamson and Schulz, 1992), it is important to assess the patient's level of depression both through tactful interview and through assessment with a questionnaire. Instruments to consider include the Center for Epidemiological Studies Depression Scale (CES-D; Radloff, 1977) or alternatively the Yesavage Geriatric Depression Inventory (Yesavage, Brink, Rose, Lum, Huang, Adey, and Leirer, 1983), because of its simple wording, its simple YES/NO answer format, and the presence of geriatric norms. We have found repeated administration of these instruments to be of consider-

---

[1] A full copy of this interview is available from Dr Sorkin, and may be requested by writing to the following address: Dr Bruce A. Sorkin, HealthAmerica, Sterling Plaza Medical Office, 201 N. Craig St., Pittsburgh, PA 15213.

Table 2. Major areas of inquiry from the semi-structured pain interview
(Sorkin, Gavlak, Hanlon, & Feldman, 1993)

CHRONIC PAIN ASSESSMENT

1 Location
2 Description of factors leading to initial onset
3 Date first occurrence _____
4 Patient understanding of current diagnosis/cause of pain
5 Description of frequency
6 Intensity (0=none; 10=excruciating)
    Present
    Usual
    Lowest last week
    Highest last week
7 Prior treatments and present coping skills
8 Events activities that worsen pain
9 Changes in lifestyle associated with pain
10 Patients' expectations about treatment
11 Patients' questions about their pain

MENTAL STATUS EXAMINATION
SOCIAL HISTORY
  Medical history
  History of psychological disorders and treatment
  Occupational and educational history

---

able help in documenting changes in the patient's mood.

Although an instrument such as the MPI (Kerns et al., 1985) contains an assessment of patient activity, it is wise to consider a scale that specifically measures daily activities relevant to geriatric populations. Instruments such as the OARS (Center for the Study of Aging and Human Development, Duke University 1978) can be considered for this purpose.

Finally, given the high prevalence of cognitive impairments caused by Alzheimer's disease, multiinfarct dementia, and other illness, it is essential to have some assessment of cognitive integrity. Perhaps the briefest and most popular tool for this is the Mini-Mental State by Folstein, Folstein, and McHugh (1980). This is essentially a structured mental status exam including items or orientation, registration, apraxia, agnosia, aphasia, and short-term memory. The exam can be administered in under ten minutes and requires only stimulus cards, a pencil, and some drawing paper.

Summary and Conclusions

The geriatric patient seen for a pain evaluation will likely present with a greater than average number of physical abnormalities. While it is important to appropriately investigate these findings, it is also important to consider the contribution of behavioural and emotional factors. The patients' coping repertoires as well as their existing support networks should be considered. The patients' psychological reactions to their pain should be adequately assessed both in interview as well as through appropriate testing. Tests should assess aspects of the patients' pain as well as their mood, attitude, and their perceptions of the impact of the pain on their social system. Specific tests of cognitive function are helpful. Norms specific to the elderly should be used for cognitive tests and perhaps affective functioning, but it appears appropriate when interpreting the scores on pain assessment batteries (such as the MPI; Kerns et al., 1985) to use norms developed from the pain population as a whole.

DO ELDERLY PAIN PATIENTS HAVE DIFFERENT TREATMENT OUTCOMES?

Although we can make some well-educated guesses about differences in treatment outcome between elderly and younger pain patients (and although as the reader might have already surmised, the educated guess is that they do not have different outcomes), the truth of the matter is that we really do not know. In theory, the matter is simple enough to study. We would randomly select geriatric and younger patients, expose them to treatment, and measure differences between them. The reality of treatment outcome research, however, is quite another matter.

Turk and Rudy (1990) described a problem in pain research that is germane to the present discussion. The subjects that we see in research studies are not representative of the population of pain patients. Non-random selection processes occurring throughout the referral and treatment chain preclude our making definitive conclusions. Only a portion of pain patients apply for services, while the rest manage on their own. Of those who are seen by a primary care physician, only a portion will be referred for treatment by a specialty pain clinic. We can reasonably assume that many geriatric patients will not be referred because of biases about geriatric patients. As noted earlier, geriatric patients are under-represented at pain clinics (Harkins and Price, 1993). Of those referred, only a portion will follow through with the appointment. Some patients will have difficulty with transportation, while others will learn that their insurance does not cover services such as psychology. Some will not be accepted for evaluation, because the clinic has an age cap. Of those seen at the clinic for evaluation, only some will be offered treatment, fewer will begin treatment, and even fewer will complete it. It would be surprising indeed if these patients were representative of geriatric patients in general. We would note, however, that this problem is representative of not only most pain research, but almost all outcome research. Bearing these limitations in mind, we can examine the treatment outcome data for older and younger pain patients.

Sorkin et al. (1990) compared acceptance and drop-out rates of geriatric and younger patients. If older patients were as anti-introspective as suggested (cf. Pfeiffer, 1977), one would predict that they would refuse treatment described as including a psychological component, that they would quickly drop out of treatment, or both. Contrary to this, older and younger cohorts had equivalent rates of treatment acceptance. Older and younger patients also had equivalent rates of remaining in treatment.

Two early retrospective studies of the effectiveness of biofeedback cast doubt on its ability to help elderly patients (Blanchard, Andrasic, Evans, and Hillhouse, 1985; Diamond and Montrose, 1983). Furthermore, a meta-analytic study by Holroyd and Penzien (1986) reported lower success rates for biofeedback/relaxation techniques with older headache patients. Later studies, however, provide reasons for optimism regarding the treatment of the ageing headache patient, and examining the unique ingredients of these studies provides insights about important modifications in treatment for the elderly population.

Arena, Hightower, and Chong (1988) reported the results of relaxation training with five men and five women between sixty-two and eighty with tension headaches of over ten years' duration. Treatment consisted of seven sessions over eight weeks of progressive relaxation including relaxation by recall and cue-controlled relaxation. Seven of ten patients showed significant clinical improvement (50 per cent or greater reduction in headache activity on the headache index, which is a composite index of headache intensity and frequency). Two subjects showed complete improvement. Patients also improved on number of days without headaches and had lower peak headache intensity ratings.

Importantly, the investigators in the Arena et al. study (1988) reported that they asked their patients to verbalize the instructions for the upcoming week. They found that many patients did not at first understand the instructions and needed additional reinforcement of the assignment. The two subjects who failed to respond to treatment reported using the relaxation exercises at a considerably lower frequency than did the other patients. This highlights the important of creating a positive motivational state in the subject and of increasing compliance with the treatment regimen. To perform optimally elderly patients may require additional repetition of instructions or more in-depth explanation of the treatment rationale.

Arena, Hannah, Bruno, and Meador (1991) reported a prospective study of geriatric headache patients employing biofeedback. Their subjects were four men and four women between the ages of sixty-two and seventy-one who had suffered tension headaches of at least thirty years' duration. Treatment consisted of twelve sessions of frontalis electromyographic (EMG) feedback delivered over a six- to nine-week period. As in the Arena et al. (1988) study, this study modified the approach to suit geriatric patients by, for example, asking patients to repeat the rationale and instructions. Four of eight subjects improved on the headache index by 50 per cent or greater. Three patients improved by 35 per cent or more. One patient worsened. Treatment was associated with decreases in the overall frequency and intensity of headaches, but not necessarily with the levels of pain seen in the most debilitating headaches. As in the 1988 group levels of use of medication did not change because of the high amount of intersubject variability, though five subjects reduced their consumption of medication by 50 per cent or more. The subjects receiving biofeedback in this study had similar outcomes to the subjects receiving relaxation training in 1988 study.

A recent study reported by Middaugh, Woods, Kee, Harden, and Peters (1991) examined the ability of the geriatric patient with chronic pain other than headaches to learn physiological self-regulation skills via biofeedback. Patients were seventeen older headache sufferers aged fifty-five to seventy-eight and twenty patients aged twenty-nine to forty-eight. These were the same patients described below in the Middaugh et al. 1988 study. Patients learned progressive muscle relaxation. Their breathing rates were counted by visual inspection, while skin temperature was measured from the right index finger. Patients also received EMG feedback with cervical or lumbar paraspinous muscles. Biofeedback-assisted relaxation was enhanced through in vivo training exercises.

Both young and older groups increased their skin temperatures both within and across training sessions, although there was no age effect or age by time interaction. Similarly there were within and across session decreases in respiration rate, but no age differences. Older patients appeared to make more rapid decreases in respiration rates early in their training and subsequently demonstrated a floor effect. Younger patients seemed slightly more likely to reach EMG biofeedback goals for reduction of cervical muscle tension. Of fourteen patients 100 per cent of the younger and 75 per cent of the older ones were able to lower their resting muscle tension levels as well as return quickly to low levels after tensing. In terms of pain reduction, older patients registered greater decreases in presenting pain and equal decreases in maximal and minimal pain.

Puder (1988) reported one of the first studies to systematically investigate the effects of cognitively based stress management in older and younger patients. The population used by Puder was unusual for outcome studies in pain. She recruited sixty-nine volunteers with chronic pain from various physicians' offices. Thus, these were not the typical patients seen in a pain clinic, but most likely were more motivated to participate in treatment. Subjects had not received psychologically based pain management training prior to the study. Therapy was modelled after the approach described in Turk, Meichenbaum, and Genest (1983) and was provided in ten weekly two-hour group programs with four to eight subjects in a group. Subjects reported decreases in the degree to which pain interfered with activity, increases in their abilities to cope with pain, and decreases in their use of some medications and other physical treatment, though the intensity of pain itself did not change. The reported gains were stable over a six-month follow-up period. Importantly, Puder reported that age had no significant effect on outcome measures that included pain intensity and self-rated activity and coping scales.

Middaugh, Levin, Kee, Fiammetta, Barchiesi, and Roberts (1988) examined the performance of seventeen elderly patients (fifty-five to seventy-eight) and twenty younger patients (twenty-nine to forty-eight) who were treated in a multidisciplinary pain clinic. Data were collected at six- and twelve-month follow-ups. Patients were seen either in in-patient or out-patient treatment depending on the perceived needs of the patients and on logistical problems such as travel. Older patients were seen on an in-patient basis more frequently. The content of the intervention was the same for both in-patient and out-patient groups and included physical therapy, occupational therapy, and psychological services, in addition to standard medical interventions. In-patient treatment lasted three to four weeks, whereas out-patients were seen twice a week for eight weeks.

Before treatment, older and younger groups were comparable with regard to psychological testing results, the number of hours employed, and the use of medication. Older patients more frequently sought out care by physicians and used emergency room services. Middaugh et al. (1988) suggested that older people were over-medicated, given that they had comparable medication use and are known to be more sensitive to medication, but this seems somewhat speculative. In essence, both older and younger patients showed considerable heterogeneity on measures such as pain and function, but overall, the groups can be seen as more similar than different, with the possible exception that older patients more frequently used medical services.

Geriatric and younger groups had roughly equivalent treatment outcomes. There was a significant time effect with both groups showing improvement, and there was a significant interaction. Older patients decreased their use of medical services. However, this could simply reflect a problem with regression to the mean of an extreme score, and so this is questionable without supporting replication.

Summary and Conclusions

From the treatment outcome studies reviewed, one finding seems to surface repeatedly. Older patients had better outcomes when treatment was somehow modified to meet the needs of the older patient. For example, both the Arena et al. studies (1988, 1991) had better outcomes with geriatric headache patients than did Blanchard, Andrasic, Evans, and Hillhouse (1985), Diamond and Montrose (1983), or Holroyd and Penzien (1986), who reported no particular modifications. Arena et al. (1988) noted that geriatric patients frequently displayed misunderstandings of treatment instructions when first questioned. They further noted that patients who failed to practice relaxation were the most likely to fail to improve. With modifications in treatment, however, older patients appeared to do approximately as well as younger patients.

HOW CAN TREATMENT BE MODIFIED FOR GERIATRIC PATIENTS
SO THAT THERE IS GREATER TREATMENT ADHERENCE AND
BETTER OUTCOME?

The literature on treatment outcome reflects the importance of ensuring adequate understanding of the processes and rationale of treatment so that compliance with the treatment regimen is insured. Patients will not follow treatment instructions if they do not understand the treatment, if they are not motivated to practice the treatment, or both.

It should hardly come as a surprise to clinicians working with geriatric patients to find that they do not always adhere to the instructions given to them. This behaviour is more characteristic than not of other behaviours demonstrated by geriatric patients (and indeed of patients in general). The average adherence rate of the geriatric patient to a medication regimen is 45 per cent. Geriatric patients frequently and intentionally underuse prescribed medications. This is of particular import given that 85 per cent of the geriatric population are prescribed medication for a medical condition (Amaral, 1986).

When indicated, treatment should be modified for the geriatric patient. This might involve repetition of instructions, as in the Arena studies, or it might involve other innovations, such as reported in the single subject case study of Linoff and West (1982) in which relaxation was effectively modified by incorporating music. Older patients, even when they have understood the treatment instructions and rationale, may show poor rates of compliance because of low levels of perceived efficacy (Woodward and Wallston, 1987). It is important to specifically solicit patients' beliefs about their ability to successfully complete the assigned tasks and to assign tasks in such a way that success is virtually insured (Meichenbaum and Turk, 1987).

Richardson (1986) suggested a set of guidelines to enhance compliance with medical regimens in geriatric populations. The advice, however, seems equally applicable to situations involving the provision of non-pharmacologically based pain management skills. In particular, Richardson advised that providers:

- Pace presentation, task relevance, and difficulty level to the elderly patient's ability
- Increase time for the elderly patient to respond
- Increase time for the elderly patient to study visual material
- Slow their pace of speech
- Provide advanced organization to help memory
- Insure that supports are available, especially for the elderly patient living alone
- Nurture patient's hope in medical care and treatment   .
- Arrange for home visits, involvement of significant others, and support groups where appropriate

CONCLUSIONS

There is a common perception that older persons have particular personality characteristics, cognitive limitations, or physical maladies that make them inappropriate for rehabilitation treatment for chronic pain. But are older individuals different from younger individuals in systematic and meaningful ways? The question is important because to the extent that they are different, treatment should be modified, and to the extent that they are similar, we can have faith that the multitude of studies about chronic pain will apply to them. We can answer the question posed in this paragraph by paraphrasing the title of our previous publication (Sorkin et al., 1990), 'Chronic pain in old and young patients: Differences *(mostly)* appear less important than similarities.' Our review of the literature on differences in coping with stress suggests that there are few differences in the two populations regarding the relationship between stress, support, coping, and symptoms. In other words, both older and younger patients find the disability associated with pain to be depressing. Both find social support to be comforting. Nevertheless, the *nature* of the stresses encountered differs for these groups. To use a computer analogy, the program is the same, but the input varies. Older people are more frequently retired and are not expected to be working. They are frequently poorer, their spouses, friends, and siblings die more often, and the elderly are more frequently ill. The different life experiences experienced by the elderly will necessarily be reflected in the content and process of treatment. Although the elderly patient will be seen within the context of a pain management program, the therapist will need to feel comfortable discussing exit events and helping the elderly patient integrate coping skills into an overall therapeutic approach.

Treatment for the elderly pain patient is substantially the same as treatment for the younger pain patient. Still, one should be cognizant of the importance of simplification of instructions, clarity of communication, organization of material, and involvement of existing social supports. It is appropriate to add some specific tests for cognitive screening and to use relevant norms for depression and activity levels, but, as with the similarity of treatment approaches, one should have confidence that norms for instruments assessing pain will apply to the older patient.

There is reason for the clinician working with the geriatric patient experiencing pain to have optimism about the potential effects of treatment. With some modifications, even patients with extremely long-standing problems can be helped to live more productive lives, be less impaired, experience less pain, and perhaps even demonstrate reversals of cognitive impairments mistakenly presumed to reflect dementia.

To paraphrase a *Yogi Berraism*, 'Older patients never had half the problems they had.' Older individuals probably were never as 'pathetic' as they had been made out to be. Not only that, but the geriatric population of today is no longer the geriatric population of yesterday. Subjects from the Baltimore Longitudinal Study (McCrae, 1982) who had originally been in the thirty-year-old cohort are now in the sixty-year-old cohort. Jerry Garcia, Charlie Watts, and Timothy Leary would all qualify as 'older' subjects in the headache study of Diamond and Montrose (1983). The change in the characteristics of the elderly cohort brings with it greater empowerment.

The popular media from *The Golden Girls* to the new Diet Coke™ commercials all portray today's geriatric citizen as vibrant and vital. It is essential that we, in the area of pain management, do not become what we have mocked, namely, rigid and regressive in our problem solving, by failing to notice, accept, and adapt to this change.

REFERENCES

Amaral, P.L. (1986). The special case of compliance in the elderly. In: K.E. Gerber & A.M. Nehemkis (Eds.), *Compliance: The Dilemma of the Chronically Ill.* New York: Springer-Verlag.

Arena, J.G., Hannah, S.L., Bruno, G.M., & Meador, K.J. (1991). Electromyographic biofeedback training for tension headache in the elderly: A prospective study. *Biofeedback and Self-Regulation, 16,* 379–90.

Arena, J.G., Hightower, N.E., & Chong, G.C. (1988). Relaxation therapy for tension headache in the elderly: A prospective study. *Psychology and Aging, 3,* 96–8.

Blanchard, E.B., Andrasik, F., Evans, D.D., & Hillhouse, J. (1985). Biofeedback and relaxation treatments for headache in the elderly: A caution and a challenge. *Biofeedback and Self-Regulation, 10,* 69–73.

Brattberg, G., Mats, T., & Anders, W. (1989). The prevalence of pain in a general population: The results of a postal survey in a county of Sweden. *Pain, 37,* 215–22.

Center for the study of Aging and Human Development, Dube University (1978). *Multidimensional functional assessment: The OARS methodology* (2nd ed.) Durham, NC: Dube University Press.

Cassileth, B.R., Zupkis, R.V., Sutton-Smith, K., & Makh V. (1980). Information and participation preferences among cancer patients. *Annals of Internal Medicine, 92,* 832–6.

Crook, J., Rideout, E., & Browne, G. (1984). The prevalence of pain complaints among a general population. *Pain, 18,* 299–314.

Davis, G.C., Cortex, C., & Rubin, B.R. (1990). Pain management in the older adult with rheumatoid arthritis or osteoarthritis. Paper presented in part at the Tenth Pan American congress of Rheumatology and Eighteenth Mexican Congress of Rheumatology.

Derogatis, L.R. (1992). *SCL-90-R: Administration, Scoring, & Procedures Manual II.* Towson, MD: Clinical Psychometric Research, Inc.

Diamond, S., & Montrose, D. (1983). The value of biofeedback in the treatment of chronic headache: A four-year retrospective study. *Headache, 24,* 5–18.

Downe-Wamboldt, B. (1991). Coping and life satisfaction in elderly women with osteoarthritis. *Journal of Advanced Nursing, 16,* 1328–35.

Felton, B.J., & Revenson, T.A. (1987). Age differences in coping with chronic illness. *Psychology and Aging, 2*, 164–70.

Ferrell, B.A. (1991). Pain management in elderly people. *Journal of the American Geriatrics Society, 39*, 64–73.

Fishbain, D.A., Cutler, R.B., Rosomoff, R.S., & Rosomoff, H.L. (1994). The problem-oriented psychiatric examination of the chronic pain patient and its application to litigation consultation. *Clinical Journal of Pain, 10*, 28–51.

Folkman, S., & Lazarus, R.S. (1985). If it changes, it must be a process: Study of emotion and coping during three stages of college examination. *Journal of Personality and Social Psychology, 50*, 992–1003.

Folkman, S., Lazarus, R.S., Pimley, S., & Novacek, J. (1987). Age differences in stress and coping processes. *Psychology and Aging, 2*, 171–84.

Folstein, M., Folstein, S., & McHugh, P. (1980). 'Mini-Mental State': A practical method for grading the cognitive state of patients for the clinician. *Journal of Psychiatric Research, 12*, 381–4.

Fry, P.S., & Wong, P.T.P. (1991). Pain management training in the elderly: Matching interventions with subjects' coping styles. *Stress Medicine, 7*, 93–8.

Gatz, M., & Pearson, C.G. (1988). Ageism revised and the provision of psychological services. *American Psychologist, 43*, 184–8.

Gutmann, D.L. (1970). Female ego style and generational conflict. In: J.M. Bardwich, E. Douvan, M.S. Horner, & D.L. Gutmann (Eds.), *Feminine Personality and Conflict*. Belmont, CA: Brooks-Cole.

Hale, W.E., Perkins, L.L., May F.E., Marks, R.G., & Stewart, R.B. (1986). Symptom prevalence in the elderly: An evaluation of age, sex, disease, and medication use. *Journal of the American Geriatrics Society, 34*, 333–40.

Harkins, S.W., Kwentus, J., & Price, D.D. (1984). Pain in the elderly. In: C. Benedetti (Ed.), *Advances in Pain Research and Therapy*, vol 7. New York: Raven Press.

Harkins, S.W., & Price, D.D. (1992). Assessment of pain in the elderly. In: D.C. Turk & R. Melzack (Eds.). *Handbook of Pain Assessment*. New York: Guilford, 315–31.

Harkins, S.W., & Price D.D. (1993). Are there special needs for pain assessment in the elderly? *APS Bulletin, 3*, 5–6.

Harkins, S.W., Price D.D., & Martelli, M. (1986). Effects of age on pain perception: Thermonaciception. *Journal of Gerontology, 41*, 58.

Haug, M. (1979). Doctor-patient relationships and the older patient. *Journal of Gerontology, 34*, 853–60.

Holmes, T.H., & Rahe, R.H. (1967). The social readjustment rating scale. *Journal of Psychosomatic Research, 11*, 213–18.

Holroyd, K.A., and Penzien, D.B. (1986). Client variables and behavioral treatment of recurrent tension headache: A meta-analytic review. *Journal of Behavioral Medicine, 9,* 515–36.

Jensen, M.P., & Karoly, P. (1992). Self-report scales and procedures for assessing pain in adults. In: D.C. Turk, & R. Melzack (Eds.), *Handbook of Pain Assessment.* New York: Guilford, 135–51.

Kerns, R.D., Turk, D.C., & Rudy, T.E. (1985). The West Haven–Yale Multidimensional Pain Inventory (WHYMPI). *Pain, 23,* 345–56.

Lau-Ting, C., & Phoon, W.O. (1988). Aches and pains among Singapore elderly. *Singapore Medical Journal, 29,* 164–7.

Linoff, M.G., & West, C.A. (1982). Relaxation training systematically combined with music: Treatment of tension headaches in a geriatric patient. *International Journal of Behavioral Geriatrics, 1,* 11–6.

Lipton, R.B., Pfeffer, D., Newman, L.C., & Soloman, S. (1993). Headaches in the elderly. *Journal of Pain and Symptom Management, 8,* 87–97.

McCrae, R.R. (1982). Age differences in the use of coping mechanisms. *Journal of Gerontology, 37,* 454–60.

Meichenbaum, D., & Turk, D.C. (1987). *Facilitating Treatment Adherence: A Practioner's Guidebook.* New York: Plenum.

Melding, P.S. (1991). Is there such a thing as geriatric pain? *Pain, 46,* 119–21.

Melzack, R. (1975). The McGill Pain Questionnaire: Major properties and scoring methods. *Pain, 1,* 275–95.

Middaugh, S.J., Levin, R.B., Kee, W.G., Fiammetta, D., Barchiesi, D., & Roberts, J.M. (1988). Chronic pain: Its treatment in geriatric and younger patients. *Archives of Physical Medicine and Rehabilitation, 69,* 1021–6.

Middaugh, S.J., Woods, S.E., Kee, W.G., Harden, R.N., & Peters, J.R. (1991). Biofeedback-assisted relaxation training for the aging chronic pain patient. *Biofeedback and Self-Regulation, 16,* 361–77.

Österlind, P., Lofgren, A., Sandman, P., Steen, P., & Winblad, B. (1986). Health, disorders, and drug consumption in an elderly population in Northern Sweden. *Gerontology, 32,* 52–9.

Pfeiffer, E. (1977). Psychopathology and social pathology. In: J.E. Birren & K.W. Schaie (Eds.), *Handbook of the Psychology of Aging.* New York: Van Nostrand Reinhold, 650–71.

Puder, R.S. (1988). Age analysis of cognitive-behavioral group therapy for chronic pain outpatients. *Psychology and Aging, 3,* 204–7.

Radloff, L.S. (1977). A self-report depression scale for research in the general population. *Applied Psychological Measurement, 1,* 204–7.

Richardson, J.L. (1986). Perspectives on compliance with drug regimens among the elderly. *Journal of Compliance in Health Care, 1,* 33–46.

Sorkin, B.A. (1993). Chronic pain increases reports of symptoms of cognitive dysfunction in both older and younger pain patients. Unpublished manuscript, Pain Evaluation and Treatment Institute, University of Pittsburgh School of Medicine, Pittsburgh, PA.

Sorkin, B.A., Gavlak, J., Hanlon, R.B., & Feldman, C. (1993). The pain interview form unpublished semi-structured interview form. Pain Evaluation and Treatment Institute, University of Pittsburgh School of Medicine, Pittsburgh, A.

Sorkin, B.A., Rudy, T.E., Hanlon, R.B., Turk, D.C., & Stieg, R.L. (1990). Chronic pain in old and young patients: Differences appear less important than similarities. *Journals of Gerontology: Psychological Sciences, 45,* 64–8.

Swezey, R.L. (1988). Low back pain in the elderly: Practical management concerns. *Geriatrics, 43,* 39–44.

Thomas, M., Roy, R., & Makarenko, P. (1989). Social modeling in attitudes toward pain and illness: A comparison of young and elderly subjects. *Pain Management,* Nov./Dec., 309–14.

Turk, D.C., Meichenbaum, D., & Genest, M. (1983). *Pain and Behavioral Medicine: A Cognitive–Behavioral Perspective.* New York: Guilford.

Turk, D.C., & Rudy, T.E. (1987). Toward the comprehensive assessment of chronic pain patients. *Behavior Research and Therapy, 25,* 237–49.

Turk, D.C., & Rudy, T.E. (1990). Neglected factors in chronic pain treatment outcome studies – referral patterns, failure to enter treatment, and attrition. *Pain, 43,* 7–26.

Williamson, G.M., & Schulz, R. (1992). Pain, activity restriction, and symptoms of depression among community-residing elderly adults. *Journal of Gerontology: Psychological Sciences, 6,* 367–72.

Woodward, N.J., & Wallston, B.S. (1987). Age and health care beliefs: Self-efficacy as a mediator of low desire for control. *Psychology and Aging, 2,* 3–8.

Yesavage, J.A., Brink, T.L., Rose, T.L., Lum, O., Huang, V., Adey, M.B., & Leirer, V.O. (1983). Development and validation of a geriatric screening scale: A preliminary report. *Journal of Psychiatric Research, 17,* 37–49.

Section 2

Family Issues

5

Chronic Pain, the Elderly, and Family Therapy

RANJAN ROY

Family therapy with the elderly is a relatively recent innovation. Family therapy gained enormous momentum in the 1960s and by the early 1970s was firmly established as a viable therapeutic method to treat a whole gamut of psychiatric, emotional, and social problems, the genesis of which could be found in 'faulty' family relationships. Family therapy as an adjunct treatment also gained some favour with medically ill patients and their families (Roy, 1990). It was only in the 1980s, however, that limited use was made of family therapy with the elderly, although clinical interest was evident already in the early 1970s (Cath, 1972; Savitsky and Sharkey, 1972; Soyer, 1972). Reasons for its late emergence as a practical and beneficial treatment for the elderly are unclear.

Any degree of familiarity with the family problems of the aged leads to the question of what caused the delay for family therapy to find its way to this rather vulnerable population. The sad truth is that the elderly do not always have ready access to psychotherapeutic treatment of any kind. This population tends to underutilize mental health treatment facilities because of professional barriers and the fear and misunderstanding of mental illness (Lasoski, 1986), this despite the fact that the incidence of depression tends to rise with age. However, when psychotherapy is offered to elderly chronic pain patients, they do seem to benefit from it. Hill and associates (1989) reported mixed outcomes of brief psychotherapy with six patients with chronic pain. Higher patient participation resulted in greater reduction in patients' distress, but the results did not generalize with regard to final outcome. Only two subjects reported improvement on more than 50 per cent of the outcome measures. The authors recommended a longer period of therapy.

Ouslander (1982), in a comprehensive analysis of the overlapping nature of depression and physical illnesses, recommended family involvement in the face of persistent symptoms of demoralization, hopelessness, and help-lessness. He recognized an association between chronic pain and depression and warned that persistent pain resulting in loss of function, self-esteem, and independence, complicated by fear of death often led to serious de-pression in the elderly. Loss of health, fear of death, complex reaction to bereavement, loss of social support, depression, and – increasingly – suicide in the elderly can form a vicious cycle. The interdiction of this vicious cycle requires psychological and social interventions that do not seem to be readily available to the elderly.

In a thoughtful review of the value of social support and social networks, Berkman (1983) cautioned that 'there is little evidence to support the idea that the elderly are particularly fragile and vulnerable to the effects of social isolation.' She, nevertheless, acknowledged the value of informal caregiving for the sick elderly. Issacs (1971) in a study of 280 hospital admissions of elderly patients reported that absence of home care because of a lack of relatives was the main cause of admission in two-thirds of the cases. One-third were admitted so that strain on their relatives could be relieved. Either way, the family support factor was implicated in all the admissions. These findings provide indirect support for a family-oriented approach in the care of the elderly.

The lack of attention to the psychological and social well-being of the elderly may be attributed to the common myth that need for emotional and social nurturance declines with age or that the aged do not have the necessary mental apparatus to benefit from psychotherapeutic interven-tions because of their compromised cognitive functioning. Steuer (1982) in a thoughtful review of psychotherapy concluded that psychotherapy re-mained an unusual treatment for the elderly. Good outcome data were rare, and even clinical reports on old people's experience of psychotherapy were scarce. She offered two interlinked explanations for this state of af-fairs. First, the elderly person's suspicion of psychotherapy as something 'crazy' people need and, second, their unawareness of available services at mental health centres and psychiatric out-patient clinics.

Elderly persons with chronic pain do not frequent chronic pain clinics. Portnoy and Farkash (1988) noted that 'there is thus the clinical supposi-tion, not yet confirmed, that most chronic pain in the elderly has a pre-dominating organic, rather than psychogenic component,' which is perhaps one reason for the low rate of involvement of the elderly with pain clinics. Reasons that bring the aged to the pain clinic are a matter of speculation. Research is so limited as to be of little help. Clinical observation and limited empirical data tend to suggest that exaggerated symptoms, probable psychogenic pain, and co-existing pain and depression may result in the referral of the elderly to a pain clinic. Portnoy and Farkash (1988) also took note of the destructive psychological and social concomitance of chronic pain in the elderly. Whether the elderly have the benefit of the full range of treatment available in multidisciplinary pain clinics is not known.

Turnbull (1989) identified pain as a major source of anxiety in the elderly. Chronic ill health, isolation, and fear of death were the other contributors to anxiety. He restated a well-established fact that the most common painful condition for the elderly was arthritis, and its onset created much uncertainty in the mind of the patient about future well-being. Patients were inclined to be very fearful of their pain – worsening, and the resulting disability. Turnbull recommended specific pharmacological, psychological. and environmental interventions to reduce anxiety in this population. Family therapy was not mentioned.

A comprehensive approach to psychological assessment of the elderly was reported some years ago by Granick (1983), who examined the merit of the assessment tools used to determine the psychological status of the elderly. His conclusion was that clinical psychologists, in general, had neglected this critical topic. Among many conditions, Granick recognized chronic pain in the elderly as an area that would benefit from systematic psychological assessment.

RATIONALE FOR FAMILY THERAPY

A very convincing body of literature supports family therapy or minimally family-oriented therapy with the elderly. Illness or disability in an elderly person has serious ramifications for family members. Generally speaking, the major share of the burden for caring for a sick or disabled elderly person falls on the spouse or in the absence of a spouse on the next generation. In any event, the nature of family involvement is drastically altered when the health of an older person deteriorates.

Shanas (1979) in her detailed survey of non-institutionalized elderly in the United States found that the major and sometimes only source of help and support for housebound invalids was the spouse. In a subsequent paper, Shanas (1984) analysed the changing patterns of family care of the elderly. More and more individuals over the age of sixty-five years were living alone, and middle-aged children and often grandchildren were the caregivers. Multigenerational involvement in the care of the elderly was the 'quiet' revolution 'that has had its greatest impact on those persons who have surviving parents and who are themselves grandparents.' Instead of looking forward to the time when their own children would be grown up, 'they now find themselves with new responsibilities – the care, and, often the financial support, of the elderly parents.' A sixty-five-year-old daughter taking care of an eighty-five-year-old parent was commonplace. Shanas concluded that middle-aged women were probably most affected by the emergence of four-generation families.

Greene (1989) noted that multigenerational families were increasingly common, and three- and four-generation families were the norm. Sudden illness or rapid deterioration of health produced a bewildering effect on the entire family system. Children and grandchildren often found themselves involved. Family therapy with a multigenerational focus in that situation was the treatment of choice. Breslau (1984), in his clinical observations of elderly disabled patients and their caregiver children, charted the course whereby a family tie between the patient and the caregiver was established and how interruption of this tie through further deterioration could pre-cipitate a new crisis. The strength of the family tie had implications for treatment. A 'narcissistic' tie between patient and caregiver could impede or even pre-empt 'standard methods of care.' To break the impasse in those situations family therapy might be an option.

Bishop and his associates (1986) investigated family functioning of vic-tims of stroke in elderly subjects (mean age sixty-six years), one year after the stroke. They found that family function, in the main, was unaffected. The subjects were carefully selected on the basis of their capacity to attend an out-patient rehabilitation program, which probably, in part, accounted for the positive outcome. Ratna and Davis (1984) investigated 142 referrals of patients over sixty-five years of age to a community-oriented psycho-geriatric service; 14 per cent of them reported being confronted with fam-ily conflicts. Some of the problems in other categories such as isolation, retirement, bereavement, and so on also had implications for family rela-tions. Only about 16 per cent of the patients in this series did not present any obvious sign of family discord.

Ruskin (1985) examined sixty-seven referrals to a geropsychiatric unit in a university hospital. Predictably, depression was the most common diag-nosis, and only 7 per cent had hysterical causes for physical symptoms. Pharmacotherapy was used for most patients, but individual psychotherapy and family therapy were useful in 28 and 24 per cent, respectively. Ruskin noted that 'family therapy is particularly important for the elderly patient because the degree to which the family can establish a supportive environ-ment often determines whether the patient will return home or will be institutionalized.' Ruskin, thus, proposed another very critical reason for family involvement in the care of the elderly.

Miller and Harris (1967) in a study that still remains unique investigated (a) the effects of the patient's behaviour on the family and (b) the effects of the family's behaviour on the patient. The setting was a nursing home in Metropolitan New York. All patients and their families were seen before admission by a gerontological social worker, and post-admission family counselling was a routine feature of the treatment regime. For the purpose of the study, elaborate definitions were established for 'improvement' and 'deterioration' for the patient-family configuration. Four patterns of inter-action were found: (a) As the patient improved, the family improved and vice versa; (b) as the patient deteriorated, the family deteriorated and vice versa; (c) as the patient improved, the family deteriorated and vice versa (paradoxical); and (d) as the patient deteriorated, the family improved and vice versa (paradoxical). There was a fifth pattern of no change. From a clinical point of view, this was an important paper as it was one of the first to attempt to delineate the complex interactional patterns of responses engendered by institutionalization of parents. The findings of this study may serve as a blueprint for family assessment and intervention for elderly parents and their family members when faced with critical life transitions.

The assessment of 'normal' functioning for an elderly couple, one of whom is sick or disabled, however, requires very different yardsticks than do younger families with no major health problems. This brief review suggests that family issues ranging from multigenerational to those affect-ing only the couple are relatively common in the elderly. Reasons for family intervention with the elderly are many and varied. One is that illness in an elderly person creates a significant level of disturbance in the imme-diate and frequently also the extended family. Also, with old age comes a multitude of transitions – from retirement to declining health to bereave-ments. A family approach needs to be integrated in the overall treatment plan, and various family treatment approaches or models with the elderly are examined below.

MODELS OF FAMILY THERAPY

Hughston and Cooledge (1989) recommended a significant departure from traditional family therapy that discourages exploration of past history and postulated that elderly people may truly benefit from reminiscing. Some of the key points were that recalling the past might be meaningful for people who do not have very much future left, it could be used to stimulate cognition and clear thinking, and it could be helpful in coping with present-day reality. They stated that 'a therapist will benefit from quick and meaningful rapport created with the elderly client and family through utilization of recalling past experiences shared by the participants ... Family experiences may be happily remembered and may provide an introduction to the underlying root of the problem.'

In a rather unusual study, Ratna and Davis (1984) investigated the benefits of a twenty-four-hour crisis intervention program for elderly psychiatric patients living at home. Their intervention occurred in the larger social context of the patient, which included the family. Usually, a life change event precipitated the crisis. Many of the events reported by Ratna and Davis, such as, illness, retirement, and bereavement, could be construed as normally occurring events in the aged. However, the family-oriented crisis intervention for the elderly did not prove more effective in reducing institutionalization than did other services. This finding led the authors to devise policies aimed at early diagnosis and pre-crisis intervention.

Benbow and her colleagues (1990) in their description of family therapy regarded the life-cycle issues of the elderly as critical. Their contention was that the life cycle of the elderly did not terminate with retirement, rather some of the most difficult transitions occurred subsequently. Two cases were presented with the purpose of illustrating the centrality of life-cycle matters in the assessment and treatment of the aged and their families. Cohen (1982) presented two cases of family treatment involving elderly persons with cancer. She used Minuchin's 'structural' approach for family treatment. Recognizing cancer as a special crisis for the family, she broadened the conceptual base by taking into account specific family life-cycle issues and coping strategies. The cases, presented with great conceptual clarity, demonstrated some of the critical issues of family therapy with the sick and dying elderly and discussed in detail the actual process of family treatment – a rare occurrence in the family therapy literature with the aged. A theoretical model for family intervention, a well-defined population, and attention to the therapeutic challenges of working with cancer patients and their families made this paper into a very important contribution to the literature.

Viney, Benjamin, and Preston (1988) proposed a 'constructivist' model of family therapy with the elderly. 'Personal construct' meant personal interpretation of events. The model posited that (a) 'families build up a system of constructs, through which they interpret their own behaviour and that of the others outside the family'; (b) developmental psychology is a psychology of changing experience; (c) family development occurs through a process of interpretation and reinterpretation described as serial recon-struction; and (d) integration of these interpretations is the primary task of development for the family. The therapeutic value to the elderly for devel-oping their own constructs in the course of family therapy is demonstrated through several case illustrations.

On closer examination, the 'models' for family therapy with the aged neither differ fundamentally from the basic premises of systemic family therapy with other age groups nor add to it. Multigenerational family therapy is very much a part of mainstream family treatment. Life change and transitional issues are at the heart of traditional family therapy, and their incorporation into family treatment of the aged is not only logical, but clinically unavoidable. Family crisis intervention is desirable irrespec-tive of age. A true departure from traditional family therapy was the notion of giving 'reminiscing' a place of primacy in working with the elderly. Even at a common-sense level this is a reasonable idea. Past experiences and memories for the elderly are infinitely more significant than for their younger counterparts, and as such may have great value in treatment. The proposi-tion, however, does not represent a model.

THE AGED AND FAMILY THERAPY

There is a plethora of clinical papers on family intervention with the eld-erly. Conjoint therapy (LaWall, 1981), community intervention (Garrison and Howe, 1976), group treatment for well spouses (Beaulieu and Karpinski, 1981), crisis intervention with elderly couples (Getzel, 1982), an ecological approach to dealing with the transitional tasks of elderly families (Lee, 1989), and marriage therapy (Renshaw, 1984) may only be a partial list for family interventions with the elderly.

Some of these treatment approaches with specific groups are briefly discussed. In what must be one of the earlier and most comprehensive discussions of family issues of the aged, Herr and Weakland (1979) made the following assumptions about family therapy with the elderly. Like in all family therapy, the focus must be on the here and now, readily comprehen-sible to the elderly, and on the resolution of the problem – rather than greater elaboration of it; the approach is behavioral; and finally, of neces-sity, the therapy is short term and focused on changing the interactional patterns of the family. In short, Herr and Weakland proposed adherence to the basic principles of family therapy regardless of age.

Banks, Ackerman, and Clark (1986) described the problems of conduct-ing family therapy with institutionalized or hospitalized elderly patients.

Regularly scheduled weekly or bi-weekly sessions with family members was suggested. These sessions would focus on a wide variety of issues such as prior conflicts, problems of discharge, emotional factors of depression, and other psychological and psychiatric symptoms in the patient and family members. The authors observed that ongoing involvement with the family assured the family's support for the patient. The authors were silent on the 'method' of family therapy employed by them.

Gwyther and Blazer (1984) described at some length their approach to working with family members of dementia patients. The first point of note was the severe impact of dementia on the entire family system. In the initial stage of therapy, which usually included children, the implications of the diagnosis were discussed with the family including the patient. Any misconceptions about the disease were dispelled. The goal was to move the family in the direction of acceptance of the disease. This could be achieved by promoting 'catharsis' in family members. This period was followed by routine reassurance and support for family members which was not time-limited and which could even extend beyond the death of the patient. Family involvement in the care plan was to be encouraged. In a subsequent paper Gwyther (1986) emphasized the necessity of working closely with the primary caregiver, as the spouse-caregiver could be at risk for 'secondary' disability. She also claimed that 'mental health professionals working with older families consistently report successful therapeutic outcome.' This claim awaits empirical validation. Although the author described her work as a specific 'strategy,' the paper was a guideline for working with a specific group of elderly and their families. The theoretical underpinning of her family therapy approach was not described.

Miller, Bernstein, and Sharkey (1973) argued that denial of parental illness, often a manifestation of established family behaviour was re-enacted during parental illness, which usually prevented successful family treatment. They described elderly persons with various degrees of disability in nursing home settings, and the inability of family members to accept the reality of serious illness in these individuals. They concluded that despite persistent efforts 'to assist the family towards an understanding and acceptance of the patient's disability, family failure with psychiatric professional services was common.' Although this paper was not directly concerned with therapy, it raised the question of family resistance to change with all its ramifications for treatment.

The clinical literature on family therapy with the elderly, in the main, is weak. This weakness has many sources, the primary one being absence of a clearly delineated conceptual underpinning for treatment. Much of what is reported in the literature appears to be a matter of common sense. This judgment may seem harsh. It is encouraging, however to find mounting clinical interest in family intervention with the aged. In the final analysis the established methods of family therapy need to be adapted to address the special problems that seem to be inevitably associated with specific age groups. As will be seen in the discussion that follows, a specific model of family therapy – with some modifications – rooted in systems theory serves the elderly just as well as it does any other age group.

ELDERLY CHRONIC PAIN PATIENTS AND FAMILY THERAPY

The past twenty years have witnessed an enormous proliferation of chronic pain and family literature (Roy, 1989). The literature is almost exclusively confined to the family issues of the middle-aged patient. The significance of family issues in the etiology of pain, the role of the spouse in the maintenance of pain, the impact of pain on family functioning, and family therapy for chronic pain patients have been the subjects of clinical and research interest (Roy, 1989). Elderly chronic pain patients and their families, as noted earlier, are almost completely ignored in the literature. The bits of information that do exist suggest that there is considerable strife in the lives of elderly chronic pain patients.

Roy (unpublished), in a pilot project of family functioning of nine consecutive elderly chronic pain patients aged sixty-five and over attending a pain clinic, and their spouses, found telling evidence of dysfunction in many aspects of their family life. The Family Adaptability and Cohesion Evaluation Scale (FACES 111) was used to assess family functioning (Olson, Portnoy, and Lavee, 1985). All nine couples completed this questionnaire. On the Family Adaptability Scale, which measures, among other things, couples' capacity to adapt to altered life situations brought on by illness, three couples were functioning on the 'chaotic' end of the scale, revealing their almost total failure to adapt to chronic pain. Only one couple was functioning in the flexible range. The rest revealed different levels of difficulty in adapting to chronic pain. The couples revealed a high degree of agreement on their perception of difficulties with adaptation. On Family Cohesion, which measures emotional bonding between family members, three couples were 'connected,' four were 'disengaged,' one 'enmeshed,' and one couple presented a combination of 'disengaged' and 'separated.' Overall, the couples' emotional bonding was somewhat less affected than their capacity to adapt to chronic illness. Again, the couples demonstrated an amazing level of agreement on their perception of issues related to family cohesion.

These findings are based on a very small sample and thus, tentative. In addition, FACES 111 is not specifically designed to address the problems of the elderly. Any generalization of the findings would be premature. Nevertheless, the data tend to confirm what is commonly observed in clinical practice. The fact that elderly patients are not frequent visitors to the pain clinic received partial support as it took nearly a year to get nine subjects for this pilot project.

Sorkin and his associates (1990) in a comparative study of young and elderly pain patients reported that when elderly patients were offered comprehensive treatment in a multidisciplinary pain clinic, their rate of refusal was comparable with that of the young. This was in spite of the fact that the elderly reported far fewer coping strategies than their did younger counterparts. They concluded that 'no data presented [in their studies] suggested that older age should be viewed as a contraindication for miltidisciplinary pain management despite negative stereotypes and greater physical pathology.' In a comparative study between elderly non-clinical Canadian and British pain clinic subjects, Roy, Thomas, and Berger (1990) reported that being single in both groups correlated significantly with depression, and widowed Canadian subjects, who had considerably less family support than their British counterparts, were significantly more prone to depression.

The above two studies furnished indirect data in support of family therapy with the elderly. Sometimes the need for family intervention with elderly chronic pain sufferers is proposed along very narrow lines. For instance, Haley and Dolce (1986) suggested that the main reason for family involvement was to educate the family members to refrain from engaging in pain reinforcing behaviours. There was no recognition, in an otherwise excellent paper, that the elderly patient may benefit from family therapy for dealing with the disruptive effects of chronic pain on other vulnerable family caregivers.

CASE ILLUSTRATION

In the following section a case is presented using the McMaster Model of Family Functioning (MMFF; Epstein and Bishop, 1981) to demonstrate the value of using a model and simultaneously to direct attention to the modifications of the model as necessitated by the special circumstances such as the age and illness of the patient.

The following case illustration was originally reported by Roy (1990) and significant parts are reproduced here. It tells the story of an 'young-elderly' man with chronic pain which had a profound effect on family functioning and challenged prevailing wisdom about the 'normal' or 'effective' functioning of a family. Family, or in this instance couple, therapy resulted in significant modification in the relationship.

Mr J, a retired civil servant, had been a patient at a pain clinic for several years. He had a long history of suffering with herpes zoster, idiopathic back pain, chronic emphysema, and periodic episodes of clinical depression.

During a conjoint session, Mrs J reported that their marriage had a checkered history. She attributed the marital difficulties to Mr J's chronically poor health. Apparently his poor health had not interfered with his career, and he retired as a senior civil servant. In addition to Mr J's health problems, they had a twenty-year-old daughter with Down's syndrome who lived at home, and both parents were very concerned about her future living arrangements in view of their advancing years. Obtaining information about this family presented a real challenge as Mrs J was most resistant and defensive, and Mr J seemed content to leave matters in her hands. On occasions when he did attempt to volunteer information, he was sharply rebuked by his wife.

The slow and disconnected history of the marriage that was elicited showed conflict almost from the beginning. Both parents had unresolved guilt over the birth of their intellectually limited child, but Mrs J expressed deep feelings of recrimination towards her husband. During the early years of the marriage, she received little support in raising the children and managing the family, and her feelings of resentment were still evident after all this time. Mr J's peripheral role in the family was explained away by Mrs J on the basis of his poor health. At the point of their inception into the pain clinic, their relationship had a nurse–patient quality.

Assessment of Couple Functioning

The problems presented by the Js will be briefly reviewed on the basis of the MMFF. The MMFF identifies six dimensions of family functioning: (a) problem solving; (b) communication; (c) roles; (d) affective responsiveness; (e) affective involvement; and (f) behaviour control. Each of these functions will be briefly described to assess the Js' level of effectiveness.

Problem Solving
Problem solving preserves the family's ability to solve problems at a level
that maintains effective family functioning. Problem solving involves seven
steps, namely, problem identification, communication of the problem to
the appropriate persons, development of alternative actions, decision on
one alternative action, performance of the action, monitoring the action,
and evaluation of the success of the action.

On a realistic basis, Mr and Mrs J did not have that many problems.
Their day-to-day existence was routinized, and their needs were few. Investigation revealed that the problems they did have were solved without
much difficulty, which is the hallmark of an effectively functioning family.
There was , however, one point of note. Mrs J was primarily responsible
for resolving the problems. This pattern had emerged over many years,
and it was not a contentious issue between them. Mr J was actually pleased
and relieved that he was not burdened with the responsibility of making
decisions.

The key question from the perspective of the chronic sick role is whether
or not Mr J was sick and disabled to the point of having to abdicate all his
responsibilities or whether he could still participate in decision-making
activities had he wanted to. The reality, however, was that Mrs J did a
remarkably good job and saw no purpose in communicating the problems
with anyone else. On the basis of the MMFF, this couple certainly did not
follow all the steps and on that basis they could be described as 'ineffective'
in the area of problem solving. At a clinical level there was very little
evidence of any difficulty with the Js in the realm of problem solving.

Communication
Communication constitutes exchange of information between family members. The MMFF proposes assessing communication on two fronts, first,
the directness of the communication and, second, the clarity of it. The Js
did not say very much to each other. Mr J was very reluctant to voice his
complaints about aches and pains, and Mrs J refrained from saying much,
lest she should complain about things that could not be changed. She
added that she was very comfortable with the way they lived and that
nothing much bothered her any more. They cared about each other, but
the fact remained that the actual quantity of communication was meager.
Their communication, to the extent that it existed, was clear and direct,
but much remained unsaid. The overall pattern of communication was far
from ideal, but was it ineffective? That is a moot question. Does the quantity of communication decline with age? How do family members adapt
their communication to chronic illness in one member? Were the Js justi-

fied in maintaining their silence on matters that could not be changed? Perhaps not entirely.

Roles
Roles are repetitive patterns of behaviour by which individuals fulfill necessary family functions. In the context of chronic illness, role-related issues assume great complexity. Abrogation of certain roles is necessitated by the illness. Can families continue to function at an effective level despite chronic illness? The role functioning of the Js was seriously distorted. As the following assessment will show, however, under their special circumstances they might be deemed to be functioning quite effectively. The MMFF examines roles on the basis of (a) provision of resources, (b) nurturance and support, (c) adult sexual gratification, (d) personal development, and (e) maintenance and management of the family system.

Provision of resources. The Js were financially well off, and they had no problem meeting their basic needs and more.

Nurturance and support. Mr J received constant reassurance from his wife about the state of his health. She was indeed the major provider of nurturance and support. He often verbalized his appreciation which was his way of being supportive of his wife. Both partners demonstrated much caring for their daughter.

Adult sexual gratification. Sexual activity had ceased relatively early in Mr J's illness. They agreed that sex did not have a high priority in their marriage, and its cessation was not a matter of concern to them. However, a distinction should be made between voluntary cessation of sexual activities and cessation imposed by disease and disability.

Personal development. The major task of the Js was to adapt to the stress of living with a painful chronic condition and their advancing years. If acceptance of misfortune and ill health was to be equated with growth, then this couple undoubtedly provided ample evidence of growth. Mrs J's adoption of the wife-caretaker role and Mr J's adaptation to the chronic sick role may be construed as desirable and even necessary. Mr J, however, probably adapted too well to the chronic sick role.

Maintenance and management of the family system. This function includes a number of tasks such as leadership, decision making, and boundary and membership functions. These functions were almost entirely within the domain of Mrs J's responsibility. The couple failed to recognize any difficulties in this area, nor did they have any feelings of inequity. Either Mrs J assumed responsibilities in this critical area of family life, or they would remain mostly unfulfilled, jeopardizing the survival of this family. Their lives were governed by routine. This couple also had the means to hire a housekeeper to lessen Mrs J's load, but she just did not see the need for that. Were the Js effective in their role performance? On the basis of the MMFF, they would seem to be in the ineffective range. However, when due attention is given to the special situation of this couple, their functioning, while far from ideal and with room for improvement in some areas, was such that it kept them functioning at an adequate level. All the necessary functions were met.

Affective responsiveness. This particular dimension is concerned with the family's ability to express a whole range of emotions. Welfare emotions denote joy, love, and happiness, and emergency emotions may be anger or sadness. The Js expressed very little in the way of emergency *or* welfare emotions. They did not express anger or sadness. They knew that they loved each other, and they had little need to verbalize their feelings. The dilemma here is about the effectiveness of the Js in their ability to express the whole range of emotions. Long years of living together in itself may not eliminate the desire to express feelings, but when the picture is further complicated by chronic illness, then affective responsiveness may indeed be compromised. Yet, they acknowledged their love for each other, and they refrained from any outburst of anger or mutual recrimination. Given their situation, could it be that their functioning was more in the effective rather than the ineffective range?

Affective involvement. The nature of family members' involvement with each other is the concern of this dimension. Lack of involvement, involvement devoid of feelings, narcissistic involvement, empathic involvement, overinvolvement, and symbiotic involvement are the six types identified by the MMFF. Empathic involvement seemed to be the closest approximation of the Js' pattern of affective involvement, despite the early difficulties in this marriage and Mr J's apparently peripheral role. His illness and retirement had thrown them together in an unpredictable way. The clinical observation was that both of them had found new ways of relating to each other which improved the quality of their relationship. There was some evidence that Mrs J was somewhat overinvolved with, and overprotective of, her husband – not an unexpected finding given the status of Mr J's health. The point of note was that while Mr and Mrs J remained affectively engaged, there was an inherent imbalance in what they gave and received from each other. Clearly Mrs J had a great deal of concern about the well-being of her husband and daughter, and her husband's medical state placed great demands upon her. An argument could be made that under such circumstances, the concept of overinvolvement is not truly apt.

Behaviour control. This final area of family function is concerned with the patterns adopted by families to handle behaviours in relation to physically dangerous situations, situations that involve the meeting and expressing of psychobiological needs and drives, and situations involving interpersonal socializing behaviour between family members and outside the family. Four patterns of behaviour control are identified: rigid, flexible, laissez faire, and chaotic. Flexible patterns are the most desirable and chaotic ones the least.

The Js presented the rigid pattern. Mrs J had almost total responsibility for fulfilling the needs in all three areas. Mr J was mostly comfortable with this arrangement, but some of the rules were too strict even for him. Simply put, Mrs J was overprotective of her husband, an issue that became the focal point of couple therapy. Mrs J made the rules, which were designed to maintain daily routine. She alone maintained contact with the outside world.

Flexibility may be an easy prey in a family harbouring one chronically sick and another intellectually compromised person. Mrs J, almost single-handedly kept this family functioning, and she devised rules that enabled this family to function almost at the optimum level. Evidently, some of the rules were too rigid even for Mr J's liking. For example, he was forbidden to leave home on his own to go for short walks or to the corner store to get a newspaper.

Treatment issues. The first and most important question posed by this case was, how well was the couple functioning? They were not perturbed by their relationship. They had slipped into a routine. Mrs J executed her responsibilities stoically and with a great degree of efficiency. Their unquestioning acceptance of 'fate' was remarkable. They fell short, in many respects, of 'effective' functioning according to the MMFF, but in view of their circumstances, they provided evidence of more than adequate adaptation. It is noteworthy that this couple had not enjoyed a particularly close relationship in the early years of marriage. Circumstances had pushed them together, and they seemed to recognize that their marriage was probably better now than ever.

So, the idea of marital therapy seemed absurd to Mrs J. She was ready to reject any such 'silly notion' out of hand. Fortunately, Mr J had a somewhat different view. He felt overprotected by her. He could not even go out to buy a newspaper. He would have liked to help her with minor household chores; he certainly was able to give her a hand in balancing the books. She would have none of it. His stress level should be kept low, she said. This difference of opinion proved very useful in persuading Mrs J to consider meeting a few times for conversations.

The couple were encouraged to discuss their relative positions on Mr J's ability to do things. This approach led to an unexpected development; these two people were, in fact, negotiating on very important matters. They were surprised by their hidden ability to openly disagree, without unduly upsetting each other. Mrs J could even express some of her anger and frustration about her lot in life, and to her considerable surprise she found her husband in agreement with her. He acknowledged that he had not fully participated in the life of this family and that he had some regrets about that. His health had placed an undue burden on her. Affective communication between them improved at great pace.

The conflicts were apparently role-related. But underneath, Mr J wanted to make amends. At a practical level, he wanted to feel useful and autonomous. Mrs J was afraid for him. Through short-term behaviorally oriented couple treatment based on the McMaster Model, Mr and Mrs J were encouraged to agree on a set of problems. The main goal of therapy was to enable the couple to share their feelings without fear of recrimination and to help Mr J to increase his level of activities. Mr J had to be less of a patient, and Mrs J less of a nurse.

Within very few weeks, Mr J reported marked improvement in his functional abilities. He was venturing out of the house and going for longer and longer walks. His wife was more willing to accept his help around the house, and their level of intimacy was beginning to improve. They even talked more. Quite remarkably, Mr J raised the possibility of resuming sexual relations, an idea totally unacceptable to Mrs J. This couple was seen in follow-up for many years. The general quality of their marriage seemed to improve with time, and in their relatively late stage in life, their marital relationship was better than ever. Quality and quantity of communication improved, their roles were marginally more flexible, their affective involvement was leaning more in the direction of empathic, and even their behaviour control seemed less rigid – not an insubstantial achievement for any couple. At the time of writing Mr J had become quite disabled, and their daughter had died, but the couple continued to maintain a great sense of connectedness with each other.

Historically a bad marriage, old age, and a very painful chronic pain condition would seem to be a deadly combination even to consider marital therapy. Were the Js the exception to the general rule, or is it possible that given the opportunity for therapy combined with motivation for change, age and even chronic pain are not insurmountable obstacles?

CONCLUSIONS AND SUMMARY

Family therapy with the elderly chronic pain sufferer remains in the innovative stages. Its use to date has been limited, and any formal evaluation of its efficacy for treatment of chronic pain is yet to be undertaken. This last point applies to family therapy with the elderly in general. An extensive literature search failed to yield any outcome studies. Yet, common sense would persuade us that the secondary family issues arising out of illness in an elderly member may have serious consequences. The question of 'burden' on the well spouse in particular as well as on other family members in general should be sufficient ground for considering a family approach. But that is only one very important reason for undertaking family therapy. The Js' case was illustrative to some degree of the larger benefits that might accrue from couple therapy. Couple treatment improved not only certain aspects of their relationship, but improved the overall functioning of the patient. This last point is often lost in the family therapy literature, namely, that the elderly patient's functional capacity can be enhanced by family therapy. Again, empirical validation is awaited.

Elderly chronic pain patients tend to be infrequent users of pain clinics, or at least that seems to be the general impression. Repeated efforts to collect data on this population by this author at his pain clinic have not yielded much result. This may be an uncommon experience.

However, the same observation has been made by others. The fact remains that chronic illness in the elderly abounds, and this literature review has brought to the fore that family therapy is, if at all, sparingly applied with the elderly chronic pain patients and their family members. The principal reasons for that appear to be (a) underestimation of family issues of the elderly and (b) perceived inability of the elderly to benefit from psychotherapy of any kind. These perceptions are indicative of inadequate understanding of the problems of the elderly, and they should be rejected. In the meantime, the plea is that the clinicians engaged in working with chronic pain patients must ensure that age is not used to deny anyone the benefits of family therapy or any other kind of psychotherapy.

REFERENCES

Banks, M., Ackerman, R., & Clark, E. (1986). Elderly women in family therapy. *Women in Therapy*, *5*, 107–16.

Beaulieu, E., & Karpinski, J. (1981). Group treatment of elderly with ill spouses. *Social Casework*, *62*, 551–7.

Benbow, S., Egan, D., Marriot, A., and Tregay, K., et.al. (1990). Using the family life cycle with later life families. *Journal of Family Therapy*, *12*, 321–40.

Berkman, L. (1983). The assessment of social networks and social support in the elderly. *Journal of the American Geriatric Society*, *31*, 743–9.

Bishop, D., Epstein, N., Keitner, G., Miller, I., & Srinivasan, S. (1986). Stroke: Morale, family functioning, health status, and functional capacity. *Archives of Physical and Medical Rehabilitation*, *67*, 84–7.

Breslau, L. (1984). Ties to family and the need for geriatric care. *Journal of Geriatric Psychiatry*, *17*, 189–201.

Cath, S. (1972). The geriatric patient and his family: The institutionalization of a parent – A nadir of life. *Journal of Geriatric Psychiatry*, *5*, 25–46.

Cohen, M. (1982). In the presence of your absence: The treatment of older families with a cancer patient. *Psychotherapy: Research and Practice*, *19*, 453–60.

Epstein, N., & Bishop, D. (1981). Problem-centered systems therapy for the family. In: A. Gurman & D. Kniskern (Eds.), *Handbook of Family Therapy*. New York: Brunner/Mazel, 444–82.

Garrison, J., & Howe, J. (1976). Community intervention with the elderly: A social network approach. *Journal of the American Geriatric Society*, *24*, 329–33.

Getzel, G. (1982). Helping elderly couples in crisis. *Social Casework*, *63*, 515–21.

Granick, S. (1983). Psychologic assessment technology for geriatric practice. *Journal of the American Geriatric Society*, *31*, 728–42.

Greene, R. (1989). A life-system approach to understanding parent–child relationships in aging families. *Journal of Psychotherapy and Family*, *5*, 57–69.

Gwyther, L. (1986). Family therapy with older adults. *Generations*, *10*, 42–5.

Gwyther, L., & Blazer, D. (1984). Family therapy and the dementia patient. *American Family Physician*, *29*, 149–56.

Haley, W., & Dolce, J. (1986). Assessment and management of chronic pain in the elderly. *Clinical Gerontologist*, *5*, 435–55.

Herr, J., & Weakland, J. (1979). *Counselling Elders and Their Families: Practical Techniques for Applied Gerontology.* New York, NY: Springer.

Hill. D., Beutler, L., & Daldrup, R. (1989). The relationship of process to outcome in brief experiential psychotherapy for chronic pain. *Journal of Clinical Psychology, 45,* 951–7.

Hughston, G., & Cooledge, N. (1989). The life review: An under utilized strategy for systemic family intervention. *Journal of Psychotheropy and Family, 5,* 47–55.

Isaacs, B. (1971). Geriatric patients: Do their families care? *British Medical Journal, 4,* 282–6.

Lasoski, M. (1986). Reasons for low utilization of mental health services by the elderly. *Clinical Gerontologist, 5,* 1–18.

La Wall, J. (1981). Conjoint therapy of psychiatric problems in the elderly. *Journal of the American Geriatric Society, 29,* 89–91.

Lee, T. (1989). An ecological view of aging: Luisa's plight. *Journal of Gerontological Society Week, 14,* 175–190.

Miller, M., Bernstein, H., & Sharky, H. (1973). Denial of parental illness and maintenance of family homeostasis. *Journal of the American Geriatric Society, 21,* 278–85.

Miller, M., & Harris, A. (1967). The chronically ill aged: Paradoxical patient family behavior. *Journal of the American Geriatric Society, 15,* 480–95.

Minuchin, S. (1974). *Families and Family Therapy.* Cambridge, MA: Harvard University Press.

Olson, D., Portnoy, J., & Lavee, Y. (1985). Family Assessment Measure. St Paul, University of Minnesota, Family Social Sciences.

Ouslander, J. (1982). Physical illness and depression in the elderly. *Journal of the American Geriatric Society, 30,* 593–9.

Portnoy, R. & Farkash, A. (1988). Practical management of non-malignant pain in the elderly. *Geriatrics, 43,* 29–47.

Ratna, L., & Davis, J. (1984). Family therapy with the elderly mentally ill: Some strategies and techniques. *British Journal of Psychiatry, 145,* 311–15.

Renshaw, D. (1984). Geriatric sex problems. *Journal of Geriatric Psychiatry, 17,* 123–38.

Roy, R. (1989). *Chronic Pain and the Family: A Problem-Centred Perspective.* New York: Human Sciences Press, Plenum.

Roy, R. (1990). Chronic pain and 'effective' family functioning: A re-examination of the McMaster Model of Family Functioning. *Contemporary Family Therapy, 12,* 489–503.

Roy, R. (1990). Physical illness, chronic pain, and family therapy. In: E. Tunks, A. Bellissimo, & R. Roy (Eds.), *Chronic Pain: Psychosocial Factors in Rehabilitation* (2nd ed.). Malabar, FL: Robert Krieger, 184–211.

Roy, R. (unpublished). Chronic pain, old age, and couple functioning. Faculty of
   Social Work, University of Manitoba.
Roy, R., Thomas, M., & Berger, S. (1990). A comparison of British and Canadian
   pain subjects. *Clinical Journal of Pain, 6,* 276–83.
Ruskin, P. (1985). Geropsychiatric consultation in a university hospital: A report
   on 67 referrals. *American Journal of Psychiatry, 142,* 333–6.
Savitsky, E., & Sharkey, H. (1972). The geriatric patient and his family: Study of
   the family interaction in the aged. *Journal of Geriatric Psychiatry, 5,* 3–19.
Shanas, E. (1979). National Survey of the Elderly: Report to Administration on
   Aging. Washington, DC, Department of Health and Human Services.
Shanas, E. (1984). Old parents and middle-aged children: The four- and five-
   generation family. *Journal of Geriatric Psychiatry, 17,* 7–19.
Sorkin, B., Rudy, T., Hanlon, R., Turk, D., & Steig, R. (1990). Chronic pain in
   old and young patients: Differences appear less important than similarities.
   Journal of Gerontology, 45, 64–8.
Soyer, D. (1972) The geriatric patient and his family: Helping the family to live
   with itself. *Journal of Geriatric Psychiatry, 5,* 52–65.
Steuer, J. (1982). Psychotherapy with the elderly. *Psychiatric Clinics of North
   America, 5,* 199–213.
Turnbull, J. (1989). Anxiety and physical illness in the elderly. *Journal of Clinical
   Psychiatry, 50* (Suppl), 40–5.
Viney, L., Benjamin, Y., & Preston, C. (1988). Constructivist family therapy with
   the elderly. *Journal of Family Psychology, 2,* 241–58.

6

Cancer Pain: Impact on Elderly Patients and Their Family Caregivers

BETTY FERRELL and LYNNE M. RIVERA

Pain is a significant problem for patients with cancer, and this is of particular concern for the elderly. According to World Health Organization (WHO) estimates, on a daily basis over 4 million people suffer from pain related to cancer (WHO, 1990). Pain disrupts all dimensions of quality of life (Ferrell, Wenzl, and Wisdom, 1989). In a changing health care system in the United States, with the reorganization of insurance reimbursement policies and legislation, and decreased hospital stays, family members are more frequently required to provide care to elderly and often extremely ill relatives. It is estimated that two of every three American families will at some time have at least one family member diagnosed with cancer (Woods, Lewis, and Ellison, 1989). This trend has increased the demand on patients and families to manage not only emotional and other issues related to the diagnosis of cancer, but also the incidental effects of treatment and management of pain at home (Ferrell, Rhiner, Cohen, and Grant, 1991).

With advances in cancer treatment and associated technology and the resultant increase in survivorship, caregiving activities at home may last several years. It is ironic that as health care has become more 'high tech,' the locus of care has moved from the hospital to the home, and from care provided by professionals to that provided by family members.

While the family is often cited as a significant source of support for the patient with cancer, few studies have examined family caregiver roles in the management of cancer pain. Family members become active caregivers, often without the benefit of training, and assume the caregiver role whether or not they feel competent to do so (Petrocino, 1985; Hinds, 1985; Kristjanson, 1986; Germino, 1987; Hull, 1989; Lewis, Woods, Hough, et al., 1989). Family caregiving requires adjustments in daily schedules, imposes financial burdens, and causes individual members to re-evaluate their relationships with the patient (Woods et al., 1989; Ferrell, Rhiner, et al., 1991; Germino, 1987; Lewis et al., 1989; Ferrell, Cohen, Rhiner, and Rozek, 1991; Ferrell, Ferrell, Rhiner, and Grant, 1991).

Researchers have consistently found pain to be a major source of concern for family caregivers (Hinds, 1985; Hull, 1989). The impact of pain on patients and their families has been cited in the literature (Woods et al., 1989; Ferrell, Rhiner, et al., 1991; Hinds, 1985; Hull, 1989; Lewis et al., 1989; Ferrell, Cohen, et al., 1991; Ferrell and Schneider, 1988; Lewandowski and Jones, 1988; Johnston Taylor, Ferrell, Grant, and Cheyney, 1993; Ferrell, Johnston Taylor, Sattler, Fowler, and Cheyney, 1993). Patients and their caregivers experience helplessness, cope by denying feelings, and wish for death as an end to the suffering (Ferrell, Rhiner, et al., 1991). Family members caring for a physically ill person in the home need skills in making decisions, planning care, and assessing the need for care (Bull, 1990).

Despite the efforts of organizations, such as WHO, the American Pain Society (APS), the Oncology Nursing Society (ONS), and the Agency for Health Care Policy and Research (AHCPR) to provide information, guidelines, and standards about pain assessment and management, increased awareness that pain can be relieved, and significant advances in both pharmacological and non-drug management of cancer pain, there exists a void in the clinical application of this information. Physicians continue to underprescribe (Marks and Sachar, 1973; Charap, 1978; Angell, 1982; Sriwatanakul, Weis, Alloza, Kelvie, Weintraub, and Lasagna, 1983; Grossman and Sheidler, 1985; Lander, 1990), nurses continue to compound the problem by undermedicating (Marks and Sachar, 1973; Lander, 1990; Cohen, 1980; Fox, 1982; Dalton, 1989), and patients experiencing pain do not request or take the prescribed analgesics (Sriwatanakul et al., 1983; Frank, 1980; Cleeland, 1987).

The literature identifies several barriers to successful pain management including a lack of understanding about pain. These barriers also include an expectation that pain should be present, relief of pain not being viewed as a goal of treatment, inadequate or non-existent assessment, undertreatment with analgesics, inadequate knowledge of analgesics and other drugs, fear of addiction, sedation, and respiratory depression, and inadequate knowledge of non-pharmacological pain interventions (Marks and Sachar, 1973; Lander, 1990; McGuire and Scheidler, 1993; Cleeland, Cleeland, Dar, and Rinehardt, 1986; Watt-Watson, 1987; Cleeland, 1988; Hill, 1989; Morgan, 1989; McCaffery, Ferrell, O'Neil-Page, Lester, and Ferrell, 1990; McCaffery and Ferrell, 1992).

The fear of addiction has been cited as a major concern of patients, nurses, and physicians (Marks and Sachar, 1973; Lander, 1990; McGuire and Sheidler, 1993; McCaffery et al., 1990). This fear has also been identified as a major factor hindering the management of pain (Ferrell, Cohen, et al., 1991). Family caregivers' fear of addiction may actually impede pain relief for the patient with pain related to cancer.

Ferrell and Ferrell (1989) reviewed 2,985 citations in *Index Medicus* that included 'pain' as a title or index term. This review revealed that only forty-nine citations (1.6 per cent) included 'family,' 'home,' or 'caregiver' as indexing terms. Pain has also been understudied in the elderly, especially as it relates to caregiver burden and elder neglect and abuse. In a review of eleven leading textbooks of geriatric medicine, only two had chapters devoted to pain. Similarly, in a review of eight geriatric nursing textbooks containing over 5,000 pages of text, less than eighteen pages were devoted to the discussion of pain (Ferrell and Ferrell, 1992).

The need for pain research in the elderly has been identified by the National Institutes of Health Consensus Development Conference (NIH, 1986). The elderly cancer patient has physical, social, and psychological needs distinct from those of younger adults. These differences pose a special challenge for health care professionals to adequately assess and manage pain.

EXPERIENCE OF PAIN FROM THE FAMILY PERSPECTIVE

Several recent studies have focused on pain management at home (Ferrell, Rhiner, et al., 1991; Hinds, 1985; Ferrell, Cohen, et al., 1991; Ferrell and Schneider, 1988; Austin et al., 1986). Family members often fear addiction and respiratory depression or drug tolerance and lack knowledge regarding chronic pain and pain management. Therefore, family caregivers may undermedicate the patient even though the patient continues to experience unrelieved pain (Ferrell, Rhiner, et al., 1991).

Pain management has become very complex with the use of multiple medications, including adjuvant drugs, and the use of complex delivery systems such as patient controlled analgesia (PCA) devices, epidural catheters, or continuous parenteral infusions. Patients are cared for in increasing numbers at home by family members who, despite their negative attitudes to drugs and lack of knowledge about pain management, assume responsibility for pain relief. Several authors (Hinds, 1985; Austin et al., 1986; Hays, 1988) have stressed the need to educate family caregivers to manage this complex and often 'high tech' care provided in the home.

Research data confirm that in the majority of situations the family has the responsibility for managing pain for the individual with cancer (Ferrell, Cohen, et al., 1991; Ferrell, Rhiner, et al., 1991; Ferrell, Johnson Taylor, et al., 1993). Families assess pain, make decisions regarding the amount and type of medication, and determine when the dose of medication is to be taken. Family members may deny that the patient is in pain to avoid acknowledging that the cancer is progressing (Ferrell, Rhiner, et al., 1991). Research has demonstrated that the family is greatly affected by the diagnosis of cancer in one of its members, and, furthermore, the family can and does influence the patient's adjustment to the illness (Woods et al., 1989; Germino, 1987; Northouse, 1984; Lewis, 1986; Siegal, Raveis, Houts, and Mor, 1991; Carey, Oberst, McCubbin, and Hughes, 1991; Maloney and Preston, 1992). Although these studies cite pain as a major concern of family caregivers, research specifically focusing on the caregivers' role in pain management is limited.

A heightened awareness in quality of life (QOL) has occurred over the past decade. This represents an interest in evaluating the impact of treatments, procedures, and medications on the overall status of patients. A specific treatment for cancer may cause pain, and another treatment may be used to alleviate that pain, but the patient is not without risk of acquiring other associated symptoms such as constipation, nausea, vomiting, and sedation. Therefore, while the current high tech era has demonstrated how much can be achieved to advance quantity of life, it has also forced health care professionals to examine the concept of quality of life. This dual focus on quality and quantity of life issues is expressed well through an inscription on a gate in the rose garden at the City of Hope Medical Center in Duarte, California. The words are those of Sam Golter, former executive director (1926–54), and read, 'There is no profit in curing the body if in the process we destroy the soul.'

Our program of research in the areas of pain and QOL has been guided by the model, 'The Impact of Pain on Overall Quality of Life' (Figure 1) which has evolved from our work. This model illustrates the impact of pain on all dimensions of life. Pain is not merely a single symptom of illness, but rather a complex phenomenon that affects the physical and psychological well-being of the patient. The model illustrates the impact of pain on the four QOL dimensions including physical well-being, psychological well-being, social concerns, and spiritual well-being.

Methods

In a recently completed study of family factors influencing pain management, we identified the critical roles assumed by eighty-five family caregivers

Figure 1. The impact of pain on the dimensions of quality of life

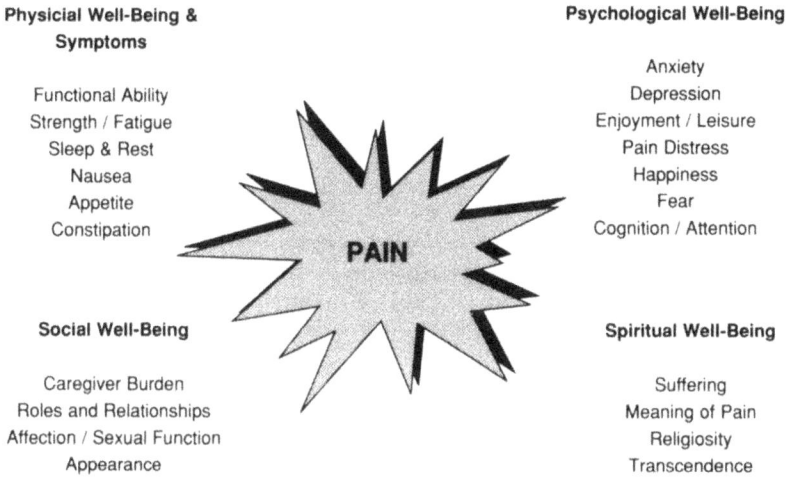

Physical Well-Being & Symptoms

Functional Ability
Strength / Fatigue
Sleep & Rest
Nausea
Appetite
Constipation

Psychological Well-Being

Anxiety
Depression
Enjoyment / Leisure
Pain Distress
Happiness
Fear
Cognition / Attention

PAIN

Social Well-Being

Caregiver Burden
Roles and Relationships
Affection / Sexual Function
Appearance

Spiritual Well-Being

Suffering
Meaning of Pain
Religiosity
Transcendence

From Ferrell, B.R., Rhiner, M., Cohen, M.Z., & Grant, M. (1991). Pain as a metaphor for illness. Part I: Impact of cancer pain on family caregivers. *Oncology Nursing Forum*, *18*, 1303–9.

in the management of pain at home. The following questions were developed for the study.

1 What are family members' descriptions of pain?
2 What impact does pain have on the caregivers?
3 What are the roles of family caregivers in the pharmacological and non-pharmacological management of cancer pain?
4 What are the primary questions and concerns expressed by caregivers about pain management?

The qualitative study utilized interviews to gain an understanding of the family perspective of pain in the specific area of pain management. The Family Pain Survey (Table 1) was developed to provide specific interview questions for gathering information about the pain experience.

Results

Caregiver Experience
The first study question asked family caregivers to describe the patient's

Table 1. Family pain survey

- Can you describe the patient's pain?
- What is it like for you having someone you love with pain?
- What things do you do related to pain medications?
- What things, other than giving medications, do you do to help relieve the pain?
- What things could doctors or nurses do to better manage the pain?
- Do you have any questions or concerns or other comments to share regarding your experiences as a caregiver in managing pain?

Table 2. Descriptors used by family caregivers to describe the patient's pain

Aching	Hurting	Sore
Agonizing	Inconceivable	Spastic
Agony	Intense	Squeezing
Bad	Intermittent	Stabbing
Burning	Itching	Strong
Constant	Miserable	Tense
Continuous	Overwhelming	Terrible
Cramping	Pressure	Throbbing
Debilitating	Pulling	Tightness
Exasperating	Pushing	Tingling
Excruciating	Radiating	Traveling
Extreme	Searing	Unbearable
Horrendous	Severe	Uncomfortable
Horrible	Sharp	Uncontrollable
Hot		

From Ferrell, B.R., Rhiner, M., Cohen, M.Z., & Grant, M. (1991). Pain as a metaphor for illness. Part I: Impact of cancer pain on family caregivers. *Oncology Nursing Forum, 18,* 1303–9.

cancer pain. Table 2 summarizes the adjectives used by family members to describe the pain experienced by the patients. Caregivers used forty-three different descriptors to characterize the pain. Interestingly, the adjectives they used are primarily sensory and are similar to the sensory scale on the McGill Pain Questionnaire (Melzack, 1975). Utilizing a scale of 0 to 100, with 0 = no pain to 100 = severe pain, the family caregivers' mean rating of the patients' pain was 70 while the patients' mean rating was 45. Caregivers, using the same 0 to 100 scale, rated their distress related to the pain at 78. These findings demonstrate the severity of the pain experience for family caregivers.

The second study question revealed that caregivers experienced severe mood disruption in the areas of anxiety, depression, and fatigue. Family caregivers reported extreme fears that the patients would become addicted to pain medications and develop respiratory depression and drug tolerance. Caregivers tended to undermedicate the patient in response to these fears. They expressed feelings of helplessness, frustration, and sadness in their inability to provide comfort to their loved ones. The eighty-five caregivers had received limited instruction in the use of pharmacological or non-drug pain management techniques and principles.

Figure 2 characterizes the family caregivers' pain experience. This experience is influenced by several factors including prior pain experiences, cultural influences, their relationship with the patient, and the meaning and understanding of the pain. The caregivers respond to the patients' pain on several levels including suffering, burden, and other emotional responses. These emotions are expressed internally through anxiety, fear, or depression, or externally through verbal expression.

Throughout the interviews, caregivers voiced their concerns about pain management at home (Table 3). Caregivers characterized the pain as a metaphor for illness and death, describing their reaction to pain as very intense and overwhelming. They reported concerns about the treatment regimens, medication usage, and addiction. Caregivers wanted to know what the future held for the patients and for themselves. Additionally, family caregivers voiced anxiety and fear about their own ability to care for the patient at home without benefit of around-the-clock professional support that is available in the acute care setting.

Caregiver Roles
The study found that family caregivers performed two key roles, administering analgesic medications and using non-drug pain relief measures, in managing the patients' pain. While caregivers expressed feelings of frustration in implementing these roles, they identified their roles as fulfilling and serving a vital need.

Family caregivers identified seven themes related specifically to the use of analgesic medications. (a) Deciding what medication to give: Caregivers reported making decisions about which type of medication to use for pain relief such as an opioid or a non-steroidal anti-inflammatory drug (NSAID). (b) Deciding when to give the medication: Caregivers reported making decisions about when a medication should be given and about the suitability of giving a medication when the patient requested it. (c) Night duty: Caregivers reported intense involvement in administering pain medications during the night. This duty was assumed by the caregivers even if the medications were administered by the patient or another individual during

Figure 2. Family caregivers' experience of pain

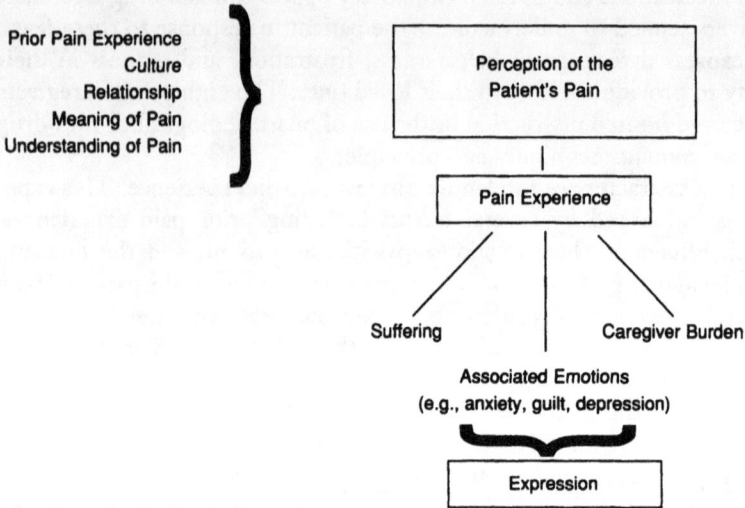

Prior Pain Experience
Culture
Relationship
Meaning of Pain
Understanding of Pain

Perception of the
Patient's Pain

Pain Experience

Suffering

Caregiver Burden

Associated Emotions
(e.g., anxiety, guilt, depression)

Expression

From Ferrell, B.R., Cohen, M.Z., Rhiner, M., & Rozek, A. (1991). Pain as a metaphor for illness. Part II: Family caregivers' management of pain. *Oncology Nursing Forum, 18,* 1315 –21.

Table 3. Caregivers' concerns about pain management at home

Concerns	*Examples of caregiver issues*
Future pain	Will the pain get worse? Can patients die of pain?
Treatments and medications	Will the treatment work? What are the dangers of medication? When and how much medication can be taken?
Addiction	What if the patient becomes addicted?
Understanding why	Why do they have so much pain? Why is this happening?
Pain as a metaphor for illness and death	Does increased pain mean they are going to die soon?
Managing at home	Can I manage the patient at home? Will the patient be comfortable at home?

the day. Caregivers reported waking up during the night to administer analgesics or to assess the patient's pain. (d) Reminding/encouraging the patient with regard to medications: This role most often centred on encouraging a patient who was reluctant to take medications. This function also emerged in relation to those patients who administered their own pain medications with the caregiver assuming the role of reminding the patient when to take them. (e) Record keeping: Some caregivers maintained written records to handle the complexities associated with administering multiple medications, decisions about dosages, and pain assessment. Caregivers reported that these records were sometimes used to communicate more efficiently with the physicians, but more often assisted them to keep track of the medications. (f) Fear of addiction: Many of the caregivers reported the role of guarding the pain medications related to their own fears or the patients' fears of addiction. Caregivers identified the need to be responsible for limiting the amount of medication used, thereby avoiding addiction. (g) Taking charge: Several caregivers described their role as one of taking over the entire responsibility for analgesic medications. They identified tasks such as assessing the pain, making decisions about medications, communicating with the physician, keeping records, obtaining prescriptions, and administering the medications. Caregivers reported taking control of all technical aspects of the use of continuous infusions or patient controlled analgesia (PCA).

Eight themes emerged related specifically to the use of non-drug pain relief methods. Five of these themes were related to physical interventions, and three to distraction techniques. The themes were as follows:

1 Positioning/mobility: Research has documented that patients tend to immobilize themselves in an attempt to relieve their pain, because movement aggravates their pain (Ferrell and Schneider, 1988). Caregivers reported using pillows and positioning the patient to provide comfort, and assisting with ambulation.
2 Massage: Caregivers identified using foot and general body massage to provide comfort. They expressed satisfaction with the comfort they were able to provide the patient through this non-drug pain relief measure.
3 Use of ointments and lotions: Ointments and other topical agents used by the caregivers were not prescribed or suggested by health care professionals but rather were identified by the caregivers themselves.
4 and 5 Use of heat and cold: Caregivers were unable to identify why they chose one method over the other. They tended to place the hot or cold device directly over the painful area and identified no formal training in the use of this non-drug method.

Table 4. Summary of family caregivers' roles in pain management

---

Caregiver roles in the administration of pain medication
- Deciding what to give
- Deciding when to give
- Performing night duty
- Reminding/encouraging
- Keeping records
- Having a fear of addiction
- Doing everything

Caregiver roles in performing non-drug interventions
- Positioning/mobility
- Using massage
- Using ointments/lotions
- Using cold
- Using heat
- Being there through touch
- Avoiding touch
- Talk and other distractions

---

6 Being there through touch: Caregivers offered reassurance through touch and their presence.
7 Avoiding touch: Paradoxically, caregivers reported that the patient often did not like to be touched or that touch caused pain for the patient. These caregivers reported feeling hurt or distressed in relation to this patient response, and interestingly, were often the same individuals who described feelings of helplessness.
8 Talk and other distractions: Caregivers reported using conversation and other techniques to distract the patients from their pain. The use of structured non-drug interventions such as guided imagery, progressive relaxation, breathing techniques, or other detailed techniques were not used by the patients and their caregivers. Caregivers reported using non-drug interventions on a trial-and-error basis. In addition, the use of these methods was almost never related to formal teaching provided by health care professionals. A summary of family caregiver roles related to pain management is presented in Table 4.

Caregiver Questions and Concerns
Two questions were used to gather information pertaining to the questions and concerns of the caregivers (Table 5). The first question was 'What things do you think doctors or nurses could do to better relieve the pain?' Five themes emerged: being there and offering hope; explaining symptoms

Table 5. Family caregivers' questions and concerns regarding pain

WHAT DOCTORS AND NURSES CAN DO TO MAKE PAIN BETTER

Be there/offer hope
'Don't give up ... get him the help he needs.'
'I hope they help with the pain as it gets worse.'
'As tough as it is for doctors and the nurses ... show more emotion and attachment.'

Explain
'The doctor just prescribes, but the nurse explains.'
'The doctors are telling me what's causing the pain. I don't know what's happening.'
'Sometimes they write it all down, which helps.'

Be honest and listen
'The doctors should be honest and not give hope when there isn't any.'
'If nothing can be done, tell the patient so.'
'Listen to what the patient tells you.'
'Listen to the family.'

Address addiction concern
'Assure the patients that they aren't going to be dope addicts. She can have two pills, but she is so afraid of becoming addicted that she only takes one.'
'Give medications that are stronger, to help [the pain].'

Giving medication
'Give the proper pain medicine. Sometimes they under- or overprescribe. It's a tightrope walk.'
'Medications are given every hour. I need some rest, something to last longer to relieve the pain.'
'... I see her clutching the grabbing my clothing. Why not give her enough to make her comfortable?'

ISSUES RELATING TO

Concerns about the future
'Will it get worse?'
'I wonder how bad the pain will get or if you can die from pain.'

Understanding why
'Why couldn't they control the pain?'
'I hear there is no need for suffering – so why does he have to suffer?'

Concerns about death
'I know he won't get better. We have to face death sooner or later. I avoid talking about it.'
'I worry about the end.'

Concerns about medications
'I'm worried whether we'll have enough medication to take care of it.'
'Is the morphine going to be able to control it? Will he be able to function mentally and through writing?'

Table 5 *(continued)*

Fear about what to do at home
'Will someone help me deal with things at home? I don't know what to expect. I have fears and we'll be all alone.'
'They have her feeling fine in the hospital – then one week at home and I bring her back worse than when she came in the first time. I'm afraid to bring her home.'

Adapted from Ferrell, B.R., Cohen, M.Z., Rhiner, M., & Rozek, A. (1991). Pain as a metaphor for illness. Part II: Family caregivers' management of pain. *Oncology Nursing Forum, 18,* 1315–21.

and treatment; being honest and listening; having fears of addiction; and giving more and appropriate medications. The second question was 'Do you have any other questions or concerns you would like to share about the pain?' Five themes emerged here, too: a concern for the future; understanding why; thoughts regarding death; concern about medications; and fear about what to do at home.

A MODEL EDUCATION PROGRAM FOR PATIENTS AND FAMILY CAREGIVERS

Clinical guidelines, such as those recently published by the Agency for Health Care Policy and Research (AHCPR), maintain that each health care facility must develop an organized program to evaluate the effectiveness of pain assessment and pain management (Acute Pain Management Guideline Panel, 1992). Standards of care related to patient teaching are addressed by the Joint Commission on Accreditation of Hospitals Organization (JCAHO), the National League of Nursing (NLN), and the Health Care Financing Organization (HCFA). Documentation by acute and home care agencies is audited for documentation of patient education. Reimbursement for services provided may be dependent on this documentation.

A major contribution to pain education has been the work of Rimer and colleagues from Fox Chase Cancer Centre. In one study, they identified the learning needs of patients in pain (Rimer, Levy, Keintz, MacElwee, and Engstrom, 1987) and then used an intervention study to demonstrate the effect of pain education on patient adherence, side-effects, concerns about addiction and tolerance, and pain intensity (Rimer, Levy, Keintz, Fox, Engstrom, and MacElwee, 1987). More recently, they have validated the importance of pain education related to the relief of cancer pain (Rimer,

Kedziera, and Levy, 1987). They have recognized five phases of the educational process: assessment, goal setting, selection of educational approaches, implementation, and reassessment.

Because the patient is the authority about the pain experience, effective pain management requires the patient's active involvement. Patient education enhances knowledge of pain content, helps the patient to understand his involvement in the process of pain management, and improves patient and family cooperation with the pain management regimen. As emphasized in the 'Family Factors' study previously discussed, this focus is especially important when pain management occurs in the home care setting.

A pain management program designed to include the patient and family caregivers may make a significant contribution to cost containment. In a survey of 5,772 scheduled and unscheduled admissions over a twelve-month period at the City of Hope National Medical Centre (a clinical cancer centre), 255 patients were readmitted for uncontrolled pain. Using a conservative estimate, this study determined that these 255 admissions for uncontrolled pain would result in a total cost of $5.1 million for a one-year period for the centre (Grant and Ferrell, 1992). An important implication of the findings was that patient and family education on pain management and increased use of referrals to a home care agency for follow-up of pain relief measures would decrease the number of unscheduled readmissions.

Program Development and Implementation

To address the needs of the elderly cancer patient with pain and the family caregiver, an educational program was developed at the City of Hope with funding by the American Cancer Society (Ferrell, in progress). This intervention study, Assessment and Management of Pain for Elderly Cancer Patients at Home, consisted of a three-part teaching program, namely, information on general pain concepts, and pharmacological and non-drug pain relief measures. The investigators reviewed existing materials and literature on pain management. Generally, existing educational materials were quite long (greater than forty pages) and utilized small print. The educational booklet developed for this study is eight pages long, written in larger print, and contains simple illustrations.

Study subjects were patients with a diagnosis of cancer who had an analgesic ordered for pain, and were sixty years or older. Once selected and after informed consent was obtained, the subject was randomly assigned to either the experimental or control group. The control group was provided

Table 6. Description of educational intervention program for elderly cancer patients
with pain and their family caregivers

Part 1: General overview of pain
Defining pain
Understanding the cause of pain
Assessing pain intensity
Use of pain rating scales to document and communicate information about pain
The importance of taking a preventive approach to pain management
Involvement of family caregivers in pain management
The relationship between pain and other physical and psychological symptoms
Use of the self-care pain management log

Part II: Pharmacological management of pain
Overview of pharmacological management of pain
Principles of addiction
Drug dependence
Drug tolerance
Respiratory depression
Use of analgesics, including opioids, non-opioids, and other adjuvant drugs
Control of related symptoms, i.e., anxiety, nausea, and constipation

Part III: Non-drug management of pain
The importance of non-drug interventions
Use of non-drug interventions as an adjunct to analgesics
Review of prior use of non-drug pain relief measures
Demonstration of various non-drug pain relief methods
• Heat and cold
• Massage
• Relaxation
• Imagery
• Distraction

From Ferrell, B.R., Rhiner, M., & Ferrell, B.A. (1993). Development and ·
Implementation of a Pain Education Program. *Cancer*, 72, 3426–32.

with the educational booklet. The experimental group received the educational booklet and the three-part education program. Table 6 outlines the education program which served as the experimental intervention.

The patient's primary physician was contacted by the research nurse when the patient was entered into the study and, as needed, to discuss medication orders including those needed to manage the side-effects associated with analgesic use.

The research nurse provided patients and their family caregivers assigned to the experimental group with Parts I and II of the education program. Audio cassettes, developed for this study, were given to the patients at the completion of each of the first two education sessions. These tapes were provided as audio reinforcement of the information taught by the nurse and to assist the patient and family with retention of the information. A Self-Care Log was used by the patients to document their pain experience and the interventions they used to manage their pain.

Non-drug pain relief methods were presented in Part III of the three-part intervention program. Five main categories of non-drug interventions were used including heat, cold, massage, relaxation/distraction, and imagery. There were nineteen interventions within these five categories. Written instructions were developed for each of the nineteen non-drug interventions presented. Patients and family members had the opportunity to try the various methods, and they received input regarding the appropriate use of these methods.

Involvement of family caregivers was encouraged in all aspects of the program. They were instructed in their pain management role and offered the emotional support needed to carry out that role.

Several instruments were used in this study including the Profile of Mood States (POMS; McNair, Lorr, and Dropplemen, 1971). This instrument has been used extensively in cancer research to measure tension–anxiety, depression–dejection, anger–hostility, confusion–bewilderment, vigour–activity, and fatigue–inertia. The Patient Pain Questionnaire (PPQ) and the Family Pain Questionnaire (FPQ) were developed to measure the knowledge and attitudes of the patients and family caregivers about pain management content. These twenty-one-item tools use 100-millimetre visual analogues to measure knowledge about pain medication and pain principles, perceptions, and experiences with the patient's pain, and caregiver roles in pain management. In addition, a Caregiver Burden Tool (Robinson, 1983) was used to evaluate the impact of pain management and the pain experience on family caregivers. These instruments were selected on the basis of our previous research and clinical practice and review of the geriatric and pain literature. Instruments were selected to minimize burdening the subject while measuring the multidimensional quality of the pain experience and its management.

Forty subjects completed the first year of the study (mean age, sixty-six years): 43 per cent had an annual household income of less than ten thousand dollars and 95 per cent had an annual income of less than thirty thousand dollars; 22 per cent were of ethnic minorities, with the hispanic population most predominant. The major cancer diagnoses were prostate (17 per cent), colon (12 per cent), lung (12 per cent), and breast (19 per cent). The average time since the cancer diagnosis was fifty-three months, and the average time since their pain began was sixteen months. These last figures are significant in identifying that cancer pain is endured by patients and their families for a long time.

Results

Initial analysis of medication use revealed that many of the patients were prescribed small doses of weak medications. Also of significance was our discovery that the patients were taking only 70 per cent of the medications prescribed by their physicians (based on oral morphine equivalents). Additionally, prior to the study, the majority of patients were not using any non-drug pain relief measures.

Preliminary analysis of patient outcomes, using dependent *t* tests, indicated that the pain education program was effective in decreasing pain intensity, decreasing perception of pain severity, decreasing fear of addiction, decreasing anxiety, and increasing the use of pain medications. Patients also reported improved sleep and increased knowledge regarding pain principles such as the use of medications on an around-the-clock schedule rather than on an as needed (PRN) basis. Patients and their caregivers were enthusiastic about using non-drug interventions. Heat and massage were the primary non-drug methods used, but each of the five areas of non-drug treatments were used successfully.

Data from the initial twenty-nine caregivers showed that the mean age was sixty years. The majority of caregivers were either the spouse (60 per cent) or adult child of the patient (27 per cent): 76 per cent of these caregivers were women, and 55 per cent were employed outside the home. Initial analysis also revealed significant differences in caregiver outcomes in the areas of improved pain content knowledge, decreased fear of addiction, improved used of medication doses and medicating around-the-clock rather than PRN, and decreased fear of respiratory depression.

CLINICAL CHALLENGES FOR FUTURE CARE

Data collected in these two studies strengthened our understanding of the patient and family experiences in relation to pain and its management. While family caregivers play a significant role in administering pain medications and performing non-drug therapies, and the role is viewed as fulfilling, their caregiving role is also fraught with frustrations, fears, and concerns. Nurses and physicians face an extraordinary challenge to address

Table 7. Teaching principles for pain education

- Information provided must be accurate and current. Content should be reviewed by experts in the area and pilot tested in a sample of patients.
- Teaching should be preceded by establishing what the patient already knows about his/her condition and pain management.
- Establish goals and objectives with the patient/family to enhance cooperation and compliance with the recommended plan of treatment. Information should be that which is immediately useful when teaching adults.
- Teach the smallest amount possible rather than overload patients who are already burdened by illness and pain. The patient must know enough about his/her condition to understand the rationale behind the regimen and be able to carry out the desired behaviour.
- Use a combination of education methods such as written materials, lecture, discussion, and audiovisual tools.
- Keep the teaching session brief with breaks as needed by the patient.
- Present the most important material first. For example, it may be necessary to first overcome the patient's overwhelming fear of addiction before he/she will be at all open to drug management of pain.
- The appropriate materials must be selected to convey the message/information to be taught. Can existing materials be used or it is necessary to produce new materials?
- Readability of written materials should be appropriate for the cognitive level of the patient. Generally speaking, no higher than a sixth grade reading level is recommended. A readability index should be performed on all written information.
- Written materials should be in a larger print for elderly patients.
- Reinforce written information with an audio cassette tape that can be replayed as often as necessary.
- Illustrations and written materials should be clear and concise. Avoid medical jargon.
- Repetition is necessary. Encourage questions. Ask questions. Have the patient/family state what they have learned in their own words.
- Whenever possible involve family and supportive friends in the educational program.
- Choose an environment that is quiet with a temperature that is comfortable for the patient and family. The patient should be physically comfortable to learn.
- Education must be individualized with consideration of cultural influences.

---

the fears and suffering experienced by patients and family caregivers and to provide support for their concerns.

While our first study reinforced our knowledge of the need for developing educational materials for cancer patients in pain and their caregivers, and in planning interventions to assist them with pain control, the second allowed us to implement the intervention. The three-part pain education program combined the components of basic pain principles, pharmacological management, and non-drug interventions with adult teaching principles applied to cancer patients with pain. Table 7 identifies teaching principles used by the investigators for developing the pain education program. The program encouraged the participation of patients and their caregivers and was designed to be generalizable across clinical settings.

Further research is needed to examine caregiver roles in relation to non-malignant pain and the impact of that pain on patients and caregivers, and to explore the impact of education on pain knowledge and pain relief outcomes. The efforts of professional societies, development of guidelines from cancer and pain organizations, and advances in pain research have served to heighten the awareness of health care professionals, patients, and caregivers to the fact that pain can be controlled and that the barriers that contribute to undertreatment of pain can be overcome. These forces have also helped to make the health care community and the public realize that patients have a right to demand adequate pain relief.

Health care professionals are challenged to make the relief of malignant and non-malignant pain a priority while maintaining quality and quantity of life for patients and their caregivers. Incorporating pain relief technology with the human aspect of comfort is long overdue in oncology practice in particular and in overall pain management in general.

REFERENCES

Acute Pain Management Guideline Panel (1992). *Acute Pain Management: Operative or Medical Procedures and Trauma – Clinical Practice Guideline*. AHCPR Pub. No. 92-0032. Rockville, MD: Agency for Health Care Policy and Research, Public Health Service, United States Department of Health and Human Services.

Angell, M. (1982). The quality of mercy. *New England Journal of Medicine, 306*, 98–9.

Austin, C., Cody, C.P., Eyres, P.J., Hefferin, E.A., & Krasnow, R.W. (1986). Hospice home care pain management: Four critical variables. *Cancer Nursing, 9*, 58–65.

Bull, M.J. (1990). Factors influencing family caregiver burden and health. *Western Journal of Nursing Research, 12*, 758–76.

Carey, P.J., Oberst, M.T., McCubbin, M.A., & Hughes, S.H. (1991). Appraisal and caregiving burden in family members caring for patients receiving chemotherapy. *Oncology Nursing Forum, 18*, 1341–8.

Charap, A.D. (1978). The knowledge, attitudes, and experience of medical personnel treating pain in the terminally ill. *Mount Sinai Journal of Medicine, 45*, 561–80.

Cleeland, C.S. (1987). Barriers to the management of cancer pain. *Oncology, 1* (suppl.), 19–26.

Cleeland, C.S. (1988). Barriers to management of cancer pain: The role of patient and family. *Wisconsin Medical Journal, 87*, 13–15.

Cleeland, C.S., Cleeland, L.M., Dar, R., Rinehardt, L.C. (1986). Factors influencing physician management of cancer pain. *Cancer, 58*, 796–800.

Cohen, F.L. (1980). Surgical pain relief: Patients' status and nurses' medication choices. *Pain, 9*, 265–74.

Dalton, J.A. (1989). Nurses' perceptions of their pain assessment skills, pain management practices, and attitudes toward pain. *Oncology Nursing Forum, 16*, 225–31.

Ferrell, B.A., & Ferrell, B.R. (1989). Assessment of chronic pain in the elderly. *Geriatric Medicine Today, 8*, 128–134.

Ferrell, B.R. (in progress). Assessment and Management of Pain for Elderly Cancer Patients at Home. Funded by the American Cancer Society.

Ferrell, B.R., Cohen, M.Z., Rhiner, M., & Rozek, A. (1991). Pain as a metaphor for illness. Part II: Family caregivers' management of pain. *Oncology Nursing Forum, 18*, 1315–21.

Ferrell, B.R., & Ferrell, B.A. (1992). Pain in the elderly. In J. Watt-Watson, & M.I. Donovan (Eds.), *Pain Management: Nursing Perspective.* St Louis: Mosby Year Book, 349–69.

Ferrell, B.R., Ferrell, B.A., Rhiner, M., & Grant, M. (1991). Family factors influencing cancer pain management. *Postgraduate Medical Journal, 67* (suppl. 2), S64–9.

Ferrell, B.R., Johnston Taylor, E., Sattler, G.R., Fowler, M., & Cheyney, B.L. (1993). Searching for the meaning of pain: Cancer patients', caregivers', and nurses' perspectives. *Cancer Practice, 1*, 185–94.

Ferrell, B.R., Rhiner, M., Cohen, M.Z., & Grant, M. (1991). Pain as a metaphor for illness. Part I: Impact of cancer pain on family caregivers. *Oncology Nursing Forum, 18*, 1303–9.

Ferrell, B.R., & Schneider, C. (1988). Experience and management of cancer pain at home. *Cancer Nursing, 11*, 84–90.

Ferrell, B.R., Wenzl, C., & Wisdom, C. (1989). Quality of life as an outcome variable in the management of cancer pain. *Cancer, 63*, 2321–7.

Fox, L. (1982). Pain management in the terminally ill cancer patient: An investigation of nurses' attitudes, knowledge, and clinical practice. *Military Medicine, 147*, 455–60.

Frank, R.M. (1980). Pain management and the appropriate use of analgesics. *Cancer Nursing, 3*, 155–7.

Germino, B. (1987). The impact of cancer on the patient, the family, and the nurse. *Living with Cancer: The Fifth National Conference on Cancer Nursing.* Arlington, VA: American Cancer Society.

Grant, M., & Ferrell, B. (1992). Is pain adequately controlled in patients with cancer? *Oncology Nursing Bulletin*, (May), 9–11.

Grossman, S.A., & Sheidler, V.R. (1985). Skills of medical students and house officers in prescribing narcotic medications. *Journal of Medical Education*, *60*, 552–7.

Hays, J.C. (1988). High-technology and hospice home care: Strange bedfellows. *Home Health Care*, *23*, 329–40.

Hill, C.S. (1989). Pain management in a drug-oriented society. *Cancer*, *63*, 2382–86.

Hinds, C. (1985). The needs of families who care for patients with cancer at home: Are we meeting them? *Journal of Advanced Nursing*, *10*, 575–81.

Hull, M.M. (1989). Family needs and supportive nursing behaviors during terminal cancer: A review. *Oncology Nursing Forum*, *16*, 787–92.

Johnston Taylor, E., Ferrell, B.R., Grant, M., & Cheyney, L. (1993). Managing cancer pain at home: The decisions and conflicts of patients, caregivers, and their nurses. *Oncology Nursing Forum*, *20*, 919–27.

Kristjanson, L.J. (1986). Indicators of quality of palliative care from a family perspective. *Journal of Palliative Care*, *1*, 8–17.

Lander, J. (1990). Fallacies and phobias about addiction and pain. *British Journal of Addiction*, *85*, 803–9.

Lewandowski, W., & Jones, S.L. (1988). The family with cancer: Nursing interventions throughout the course of living with cancer. *Cancer Nursing*, *11*, 313–21.

Lewis, F.M. (1986). The impact of cancer on the family: A critical analysis of communication in late stage cancer. *International Journal of Psychiatry in Medicine*, *135*, 203–16.

Lewis, F.M., Woods, N.F., Hough, E.E., & Bensley, L.S. (1989). The family's functioning with chronic illness in the mother: The spouse's perspective. *Social Science Medicine*, *29*, 1261–9.

Maloney, C.H., & Preston, F. (1992). An overview of home care for patients with pain. *Oncology Nursing Forum*, *19*, 75–80.

Marks, R.M., & Sachar, E.J. (1973). Undertreatment of medical inpatients with narcotic analgesics. *Annals of Internal Medicine*, *78*, 173–81.

McCaffery, M., & Ferrell, B.R. (1992). Opioid analgesics: Nurses' knowledge of doses and psychological dependence. *Journal of Nursing Staff Development*, (March/April), 77–84.

McCaffery, M., Ferrell, B.A., O'Neil-Page, E., Lester, M., & Ferrell, B.R. (1990). Nurses' knowledge of opioid analgesic drugs and psychological dependence. *Cancer Nursing*, *13*, 21–7.

McGuire, D.B., & Sheidler, V.R. (1993). In: S.L. Groenwald, M.H. Frogge,

M. Goodman, & C.H. Yarbro (Eds.), *Cancer Nursing: Principles and Practice*. Boston: Jones and Bartlett, 499–556.

McNair, D.M., Lorr, M., & Dropplemen, L.F. (1971). *Profile of Mood States*. San Diego: EDITS, Educational and Testing Service.

Melzack, R. (1975). The McGill pain questionnaire: Major properties and scoring methods. *Pain, 1*, 275–99.

Morgan, J.P. (1989). American opiophobia: Customary underutilization of opioid analgesics. In: C.S. Hill & W.S. Fields (Eds.), *Advances in Pain Research and Therapy*, vol. *11*. New York: Raven Press, 181–95.

National Institutes of Health (1986). The integrated approach to the management of pain. *National Institutes of Health Consensus Development Conference Statement*. Bethesda, MD: National Institutes of Health.

Northouse, L. (1984). The impact of cancer on the family: An overview. *International Journal of Psychiatry in Medicine, 14*, 215–42.

Petrocino, B.M. (1985). Characteristics of hospice patients, primary caregivers, and nursing care problems: Foundation for future research. *Hospice Journal, 1*, 28–33.

Rimer, B.K., Kedziera, P., & Levy, M.H. (1987). The role of patient education in cancer pain control. *Hospice Journal, 8*, 171–91.

Rimer, B., Levy, M.H., Keintz, M.K., Fox, L., Engstrom, P.F., & MacElwee, N. (1987). Enhancing cancer pain control regimens through patient education. *Patient Education and Counseling, 10*, 267–77.

Rimer, B., Levy, M., Keintz, M.K., MacElwee, N., & Engstrom, P. (1987). Improving cancer patients' pain control through education. In: P. Engstrom, L.E. Mortenson, & P.N. Anderson (Eds.), *Advances in Cancer Control: The War on Cancer – 15 Years of Progress*. New York: Alan R. Liss, 123–7.

Robinson, B. (1983). Validation of a caregiver strain index. *Journal of Gerontology, 38*, 344–88.

Siegal, K., Raveis, V.H., Houts, P., & Mor, V. (1991). Caregiver burden and unmet patient needs. *Cancer, 61*, 1131–40.

Sriwatanakul, K., Weis, O.F., Alloza, J.L., Kelvie, W., Weintraub, M., & Lasagna, L. (1983). Analysis of narcotic analgesic usage in the treatment of postoperative pain. *Journal of the American Medical Association, 250*, 926–9.

Watt-Watson, J. (1987). Nurses' knowledge of pain issues: A survey. *Journal of Pain and Symptom Management, 2*, 207–11.

Woods, N.F., Lewis, F.M., & Ellison, E.S. (1989). Living with cancer: Family experiences. *Cancer Nursing, 12*, 28–33.

World Health Organization (1990). *Cancer Pain Relief*. Geneva: World Health Organization.

Section 3

Psychological and Medical Interventions

7

Geriatric Pain

S.W. HARKINS, BELINDA T. LAGUA,
D.D. PRICE, and RALPH E. SMALL

The first comprehensive review of age differences in pain perception appeared in 1980 and emphasized the relations between old age and sensitivity to experimental pain. In that review it was concluded that there was no convincing evidence that pain sensibilities, at least as studied in the laboratory, decreased with normal ageing (Harkins and Warner, 1980). This contrasts with the often accepted point of view that old individuals can tolerate minor surgical procedures and even dental extractions with little or no discomfort or suffering (Critchley, 1931).

Since 1980 a considerable amount of new information has been generated on pain perception in the geriatric population. It is the objective of this chapter to present a limited review of this information and to suggest a model for the study of pain. It is also the purpose of this chapter to explore what pain can tell us about ageing and if ageing can tell us anything about the human experience of pain. For the most part, this chapter will raise unanswered questions. We hope, however, that it will serve to foster new research and thus lead to a better understanding of the interactions of old age and physiological, psychological, and social aspects of pain and, most importantly, by doing so, lead to improvements in the quality of care for elderly individuals with pain.

Preliminary answers to several questions frequently raised with regard to age and pain (Melding, 1991; Harkins and Warner, 1980; Harkins and Price, 1992) can be given at this time. These include:

1 Does old age, *per se*, dull the sense of pain (nociception) in a clinically significant manner? The answer to this question is very likely no for some but not for all types of pain.
2 Do the old benefit from standard interventions for acute and chronic

pain in the same manner as younger adults? The answer to this question is a definite yes, and specialty clinics for the diagnosis and treatment of pain in the elderly are warranted.

3 Does pain as a symptom present atypically in the elderly? The short answer is yes and no, and this relates directly to (1) above. Pain from deep structures may not accompany the clinical presentation of certain acute conditions in the old. For example, painless ischaemia increases with age and can complicate rapid and accurate diagnosis of acute myocardial or mesenteric infarct. In other conditions, such as Parkinson's disease, pain is an unexpected and recurrent problem in a significant number of patients. Nevertheless, it will be suggested here that acute pain associated with injury may not differ with age if frank involutional changes in structure are absent.

4 Do gerontophobia and ageist attitudes influence provision of health care to the elderly with chronic pain problems? The answer is yes.

This chapter is organized around issues that are considered central to current understanding of geriatric pain. First, definitions and demographic issues are discussed. Second, a very brief overview of physiological and psychosocial models of pain is presented. Third, possible characteristics of presbyalgos (presby – old; algos – pain) are discussed. Attention is also given to special issues related to pain assessment and the treatment of geriatric pain. Barriers to assessment and treatment are discussed in this context. A major orientation of this chapter is that simple pain assessment tools that recognize the complexity of the human pain experience can be effective in the determination of treatment efficacy for geriatric pain. Examples are given using a simple visual analogue scaling technique for the evaluation of pain sensation and two different forms of pain-related suffering in different age groups.

DEFINITIONS AND ASSUMPTIONS CONCERNING AGEING

Because the fields of gerontology and geriatrics are relatively new, some basic definitions may be helpful. Gerontology is the scientific study of ageing in the later years of life. Geriatrics, in turn, is concerned with clinical issues in the older patient. Senescence is the biological term for the age-related changes that occur in the later years of life that are associated with an increasing probability of death. This process of senescence is associated with well-documented changes in most senses. These include presbycusis (also presbyacusis; presby – old; cusis – audition) and presbyopia

(opia – vision; see reviews by Fozard, 1990; Olsho, Harkins, and Lenhardt, 1985). While systematic study of the effects of age on the major senses has been the subject of considerable effort, similar attention has not been paid to age differences or changes in pain. This is unfortunate because of the great importance of pain as a symptom in diagnosis and the need for its control in humanitarian care. Another important distinction in gerontology is between the young-old and the old-old. This distinction explicitly recognizes the many physiological, medical, social, and economic differences between individuals under eighty-five and those eighty-five years of age and older. It is the old-old, those in their late eighties or older, who are most likely frail, with multiple, chronic health problems. Many of the health and physical problems faced by these individuals are associated with recurrent and chronic pain. Little research to date has specifically addressed pain in the old-old.

Another issue that deserves definition in relation to age and pain is that of activities of daily living (ADLs). The ability to function in day-to-day activities can be limited by the presence of pain, by frailty associated with age-related disease, by chronic degeneration, or by their interactions. When limitations in ADLs occur because of pain, it has been suggested that the individual is at risk of suffering that goes beyond that caused by the pain itself (Elliott and Harkins, 1991, 1992; Harkins and Price, 1992a, 1992b; Price and Harkins, 1992; Price, 1988). This critically important issue, and the resulting impact of pain on limitations in ADLs, has not been systematically evaluated in the old-old.

Finally, it may be beneficial to present some classifications of pain found in the literature and in clinical settings. Acute pain is often an indicator of a physiological problem that requires treatment. It has a distinct, tangible onset and is accompanied by increased autonomic nervous system signs such as increased blood pressure, increased heart rate, and diaphoresis (Bonica, 1990; Wall, 1990; France, 1989). Chronic pain, however, lasts longer than the usual length of an acute disease or longer than a reasonable time for an injury to heal. There is often no sign of increased autonomic nervous system activity, and in a majority of cases the diagnostic work-up fails to find a source for the pain (Bonica, 1990; Wall, 1990). Acute and chronic pain are the two main classifications of pain, but there are two additional ones. Acute recurrent pain is caused by repeated nociceptive stimulus from a chronic pathological condition such as osteoarthritis; such pain may best be defined as chronic in the geriatric population (Harkins, Price, Bush, and Small, 1994). Additionally, cancer pain may be considered a form of acute pain.

The population structure of the industrialized nations has aged over the past century, and this trend is expected to continue. This has been referred to as the greying of these societies. For example, the median age of the population of the United States and Canada is currently close to thirty-three years of age, while Mexico has a much younger population with a median age of approximately nineteen years. The greying of the more developed nations reflects, to a large degree, reductions in infant and child mortality and deaths resulting from acute illness, and improved sanitation, education, and nutrition. It is not the result of any dramatic increases in life expectancy in the later years of life.

Life expectancy from birth has shown great increases since 1900 when approximately three million Americans were sixty-five years or older and represented approximately 4 per cent of the population. Estimates for 1992 are that approximately 13 per cent of the United States population is above sixty-four years of age. Projections for 2030 suggest that those sixty-five and above will represent about 22 per cent of the population. The increase in life expectancy from birth has not been accompanied by nearly as dramatic a change in increased longevity in the later years of life. That is, life expectancy from age eighty-five has not changed since 1900 nearly as dramatically as life expectancy from birth has. This has led to a compression of mortality into the later years of the human life span (Fries, 1980; Fries, Green, and Levine, 1989). Thus, while more individuals are living longer, the upper age limit of life for the human seems fixed. This compression of mortality is illustrated in Figure 1 (Wegman, 1990).

Figure 1 is based on the annual summary of deaths from the National Center for Health Statistics for 1989 (Wegman, 1990) and shows the approximate percentage of persons surviving from one age interval to the next. This curve represents what has been termed the rectangularization of the survival curve (Fries, 1980; Fries, Green, and Levine, 1989). Perhaps most importantly for the health care system, the proportion of the population age eighty-five and older has increased the most (30 per cent) from 1950. This group of individuals, as noted above, represent the 'old-old' and are those at greatest risk of frailty, dementia, and degenerative conditions often associated with chronic pain.

In addition to the compression of mortality it has been suggested that morbidity is being compressed more and more into the later years of life. That is, we not only live longer but also healthier lives (Fries,1980; Fries et al., 1989). Yet the old-old, the group that is proportionately increasing the

Figure 1. Age dependent survival rates in the United States, 1989

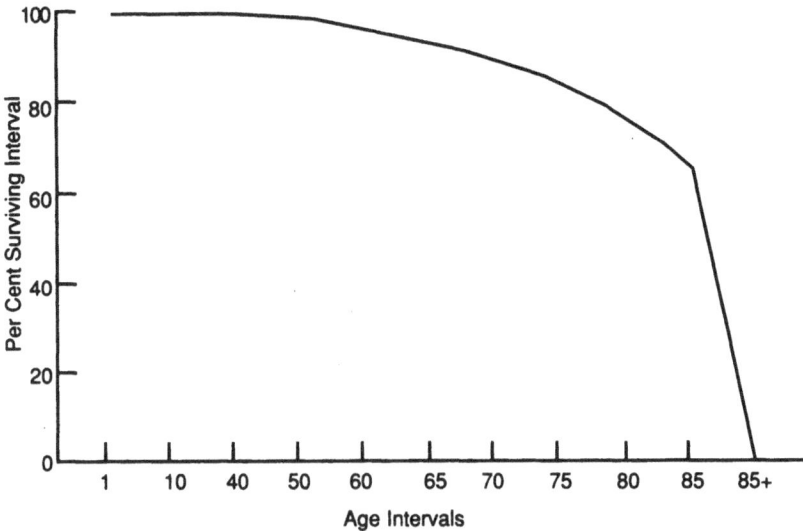

Probability of survival into the next interval as a function of age in the general population of the United States in 1989. Note that the probability of survival begins decreasing dramatically at about age 80. This phenomenon has been referred to as the 'rectangularization of the survival curve' or the 'compression of mortality' and is characteristic of the more developed countries. See Fries, 1980. Data abstracted from Wegman, 1990, *Pediatrics*, *86*, 836–47 (Table 3).

most are individuals with a significant likelihood of multiple, chronic degenerative illness, about whom there is no systematic research on pain prevalence or management. These are the individuals most at risk for significant frailty, decreasing cognitive capacity, loss of social support systems, and increasing loss of financial resources, especially for those in institutional settings with 'spend down regulations.' When chronic degenerative conditions often associated with old age are considered, particularly those associated with discomfort and pain, it may be that old age is associated with increasing morbidity.

Whether or not morbidity is decreasing in the geriatric population is a major question for systematic epidemiological research. As is indicated throughout this chapter, such research must include both acute and chronic pain, if the question of compression of morbidity in later life is to be appropriately addressed.

PHYSIOLOGICAL AND PSYCHOSOCIAL MODELS OF PAIN

Scientists have proposed various models to understand pain perception and tolerance. Initial attempts to understand pain were mainly from a physiological perspective. Later models have included the psychological or experiential aspects in modelling the human experience of pain.

The specificity model, or stimulus response model, was one of the original theories proposed. This model claimed that when peripheral sensory receptors are stimulated as a result of injury to the body, nerve impulses travel through the spinal cord to the brain. The intensity of pain is assumed to be a direct reflection of the activation of 'pain receptors.' Various treatment techniques that followed this model were effective for acute type pains, but not chronic pains (Saxon, 1991).

The gate control theory was the first model to systematically integrate sensory, emotional, and cognitive influences on pain. The theory claims that there is a type of gating mechanism in the spinal cord that controls the perception of pain at the spinal cord, subcortical, and cerebral cortical levels. Nociceptors, sensory receptors to pain found in the skin and subcutaneous tissues, are responsive to chemical, thermal, electrical, and mechanical stimulation. These nociceptors are terminal endings of either A-delta or C nerve fibres. A-delta fibres are larger diameter nerves that relay localized, sharp, pricking pains that are rapidly evoked, but of short duration. C fibres are small diameter nerves that relay deep, burning, diffuse, dull pains that persist. A-beta fibres are large in diameter and carry other non-painful, mechanosensory information. All types of nerve fibres travel to the dorsal horn of the spinal cord. From there the stimulus is transmitted to the thalamus, hypothalamus, limbic system, and cerebral cortex, where the processing actually relating to perception of pain occurs.

The gate mechanism is controlled by the composition of activated types of afferent nerves as well as by descending modulation from the brain and spinal cord. C and A-delta fibres facilitate pain by opening the gate; whereas, A-beta fibres input using low threshold mechanoceptors (touch) to suppress the transmission of pain by closing the gate. This theoretical gate can also be influenced to open and close by the brain and spinal cord. This theory allows for emotional and psychological factors to play a part in the perception of pain (Michlovitz, 1986; Wall, 1990). The selective effects of age at each ascending level as well as its effect on descending modulation have not been systematically evaluated.

Another explanation of variations in pain perception is the presence of neuroregulators in peripheral and central neurons. These chemicals are natural pain moderators which act at the synapses between neurons. Neurotransmitters may be indolamines (i.e., serotonin), catecholamines (i.e., norepinephrine and dopamine), or enkephalins/endorphins. The mechanism of action of these substances is not well understood (Wall, 1990). Neurotransmitter changes do occur with regularity in the old, but these are specific to disease processes (for example, dopamine in parkinsonism or acetylcholine in Alzheimer's disease). Neuroregulatory changes with age that may influence the perception of pain and pain-related suffering await a better understanding of both the pain and of human ageing in the later years of life.

The learning theory of pain distinguishes between the initial physiological reaction to a painful stimulus and the resultant behaviours. Respondent pain behaviours are actions that result from the actual nociception. Operant pain behaviours are actions that develop when the pain experience is linked to forms of reinforcement such as receiving pain medication, or attention, or being allowed to avoid unpleasant situations. The reinforcements encourage the pain behaviour to linger on and become separated from the original painful stimulus. If respondent pain behaviours last long enough, learning will occur and behaviours will then be controlled by the operant pain behaviours. In chronic pain both respondent and operant pain behaviours may exist (Saxon, 1991). Certainly, learning theory can contribute much to our understanding of cross-sectional (birth cohort) differences in response to stressors, including pain.

It is the psychological aspect of pain that adds complexity to understanding pain mechanisms and is an area of current debate. Pain may begin with the noxious stimulus that can lead to tissue damage, but it does not stop there. There also is cognitive appraisal of the stimulus as well as evaluation of the context in which the stimulus occurs. Finally there is the affective dimension of pain.

Recently one pain model proposed that the affective dimension of pain is composed of two stages. The first of these stages is related to the immediate unpleasantness of the pain. The second is dependent upon subsequent ramifications of experiencing pain that are strongly influenced by subject variables (Price, 1992). This distinction (see Price, 1988; Price and Harkins, 1992) is discussed in detail later in this chapter.

The literature that addresses the psychological aspect of pain primarily examines people who experience chronic pain, as opposed to acute pain. Regardless of the classification, pain that persists can inhibit the person's functional capacities, emotional state, psychological condition, and socioeconomic status. The longer a person experiences chronic pain, the more the pain is likely to affect the psychological and social factors (France, 1989). Psychological conditions that are often found in people with chronic pain include depression, anxiety, adjustment disorder, dysthymia, and personality disorder. For people with chronic pain of an organic nature it is estimated that 20 to 40 per cent have major depression and 40 per cent have dysthymic disorders (France, 1989). Furthermore, the cause–effect relationship between pain and depression may go in either direction. Being depressed may lead to higher levels of pain, and high levels of pain may cause a person to become depressed (Williams and Schulz, 1988).

In order to understand how people can develop these psychological disorders it would be beneficial to examine what factors influence the affective dimension of pain. First, consider the concept of locus of control (LOC). People who have an internal LOC believe that they can affect their experiences/outcomes by their own behaviour. However, people who have an external LOC do not believe that their behaviours can influence their experiences, but that instead it is external factors, such as chance or fate, that dictate their experiences. Research has shown that chronic pain patients who have external LOC perception of pain are more depressed than are those people with internal LOC (Skevington, 1983). In addition, LOC in patients with chronic pain is significantly correlated with the use of pain coping strategies and psychological distress. People with more external or chance LOC are more likely to have increased pain and functional impairment because of ineffective use of coping strategies and avoidance of activity (Crisson, and Keefe, 1988). Being sensitive to individual differences in personality factors may be beneficial in both the assessment and treatment of the pain.

Next, consider how pain perception affects the person's functional abilities. Research on people with spinal cord injuries has shown that the amount of distress associated with pain is correlated to the extent to which the pain interferes with expected functional activities. In fact, in a study by Elliott and Harkins (1991) comparing paraplegic patients and quadriplegic patients with similar levels of chronic pain, paraplegics perceived the pain as more unpleasant or disturbing than did quadriplegics. This may reflect the greater potential for self-care in relation to functional activities among paraplegics (Elliott and Harkins, 1991). In another study of the effect of pain associated with menstruation, it was found that pain-related emotional distress was positively correlated with the perceived interference with functional activities (Elliott and Harkins, 1992). It is interesting that the two studies yielded very similar results despite the differences in subjects and types of pain. The results were consistent in that the model of interference resulting from pain was a major determinant of pain-related suffering.

Another factor that has been found to affect a person's pain experience is social support. Overall, the presence of social support is viewed as beneficial for recovery, rehabilitation, and adjustment to chronic disease (Wallston, Alagna, Devellis, and Devellis, 1983). Research on the influence of social support on pain behaviour has demonstrated interesting results. The number of people available for support was not a significant factor, but the level of satisfaction with the support did influence pain behaviour of chronic pain patients. People who reported high levels of satisfaction with their support demonstrated higher levels of pain behaviour. The social support for these patients worked as a reinforcement to continue pain behaviours. The persistence of pain behaviours such as guarding of movement by muscles may have perpetuated the pain experience by creating muscle tension and fatigue (Gil, Keefe, Crisson, and Van Dalfren, 1987).

Physiological models of pain are not adequate to explain why pain experience varies from one individual to the next. The three factors discussed above – locus of control, interference with functional activities, and social support – are examples of psychological and social factors that influence the affective dimension of pain and pain behaviours. These examples are certainly not the limit of psychosocial factors influencing pain-related suffering and behaviour. Other examples include cognitive models, expectancies, socioeconomic status, cultural background, gender, religious beliefs, and social roles. Any of these may be influenced by chronological age in the later years of life. Furthermore, both actual and perceived social support are likely to be factors mediating chronic pain-related suffering resulting from degenerative processes in the elderly. This is likely as true in the long-term-care setting as in the community dwelling.

Despite the great advances in our understanding on mechanisms of pain, there is still no single model or schema which completely describes the nature of the human pain experience. Thus, it should not be surprising that the effects of chronological age on pain-related suffering are unclear. It is, however, surprising that many have accepted that there are losses in mechanisms subserving pain in the old in a fashion that parallels age-related losses in most other senses.

Presbyalgos?

If age has a systematic impact on pain perception then this would be termed presbyalgos (Harkins, Kwentus, and Price, 1984, 1990). Table 1 presents possible characteristics of presbyalgos in terms of possible age

Table 1. Possible characteristics of presbyalgos

Sensory Components:
Possible age effects:
- Increased pain thresholds.
- Increased pain tolerance.
- Reduced ability to discriminate between pain of various intensities.
- Reduced ability to discriminate among different pains.
- Increased frequency of atypical pain as a symptom of disease processes.
- Reduced need for analgesics because of presbyalgos.
- Reduced need for anaesthetics.

Primary Affective Components:
Characteristics:
   Strongly related to pain intensity and Autonomic Nervous System arousal.
   Related to appraisal of the present and short term future.
   Cognitive appraisal.
Possible age effects:
- Reduced unpleasantness of pain, because of reduced sensory intensity of pain in general.
- Reduced unpleasantness of pain resulting from decreased arousal, exteroceptive (sight, sound) and interoceptive (startle, autonomic) responses resulting in reduced segmental responses to painful injury.
- Reduced general aversiveness of nociceptive stimuli.
- Decreased perception of threat, distress, annoyance associated with the intensity of the painful sensation and its accompanying arousal.
- Change in cognitive appraisal.

Secondary affective components of pain:
Characteristics:
   Related to past and long-term future.
   Cognitive appraisal.
   Related to or representative of suffering.
   Not measurable in experimental studies of pain.

Stage II pain shares many properties of emotional suffering. Suffering is defined here 'as the state of severe distress associated with events that threaten the intactness of the person.' (see Text). There is confusion between chronic pain and suffering because disease models dominate thinking concerning pain.

Unameliorated pain-related suffering (Stage II affect) requires different interventions than those traditionally used for control of the sensory intensity or the primary affective components of pain.

No studies exist of the effects of age on the secondary affective component of human pain.

Table 2. Summary of laboratory studies of the effect of age on psychophysical indices of pain sensitivity

Stimulus	*Source* (Reference)	*Psychophysical end points and findings*
1. Thermal:		
A. Radiant		
heat:	Schumacher et al., 1940	Sensory Thresholds *No age effects*
	Hardy et al., 1943	Sensory Thresholds *No age effects*
	Chapman and Jones, 1944	Sensory Thresholds *Higher in elderly* Reaction Thresholds *Higher in elderly*
	Birren et al., 1950	Pain sensory thresholds *No age effects* Pain reaction thresholds *No age effects*
	Sherman and Robillard, 1964a, 1964b	Sensory Thresholds *Higher in elderly* Reaction Thresholds *Higher in elderly*
	Procacci et al., 1970, 1974	Sensory Thresholds *Higher in elderly*
	Clark and Mehl, 1971	Sensory Thresholds *Higher in 55 year olds compared to younger adults*
B. Contact		
Heat:	Kenshalo, 1986	Sensory Thresholds *No age effects*
	Harkins, Price, and Martelli, 1986	Magnitude Matching *Slight age effects*
2. Electrical shock:		
A. Cutaneous:	Collins and Stone, 1966	Sensory Threshold *Lower in elderly* Tolerance *Lower in elderly*
	Tucker et al., 1989	Sensory Threshold *Higher in elderly*
B. Tooth:	Mumford, 1965	Sensory Threshold *No age effects*

(Continued)

Table 2 (*continued*)

	Mumford, 1968	Sensory Threshold *No age effects*
	Harkins and Chapman, 1976	Sensory Threshold *No age effects* Discrimination accuracy *Lower in elderly* Response bias (criteria) *Age effects: Variable*
	Harkins and Chapman, 1976	Sensory Threshold *No age effects* Discrimination accuracy *Lower in elderly* Response bias (criteria) *Age effects: Variable*
C. Pressure: Achilles Tendon:	Woodrow et al., 1972	Tolerance *Lower in elderly*
D. Cold Pressor:	Walsh et al., 1989	Tolerance (time) Males: lower with increasing age Females: Minimal increase with increasing age

Adapted from Harkins and Warner, 1980; corrected from Harkins and Price, 1992.

effects on the sensory component, the primary affective component, and the secondary affective component of pain. Findings regarding each of these pain components in relation to age are discussed.

Sensory Components of Pain

An initial point of departure in the study of possible characteristics of presbyalgos is to evaluate the effects of senescence on the sensory components of pain. This can be done by detailed review of laboratory studies of age differences in response to various experimentally induced pain.

Laboratory studies of age differences in induced pain perception have focused on a number of psychophysical end-points including threshold, tolerance, and discrimination of pain intensity. Taken together the studies are equivocal. Some studies indicate no age-related changes in sensitivity to experimental pain intensity in healthy individuals, others indicate a decrease in sensory acuity, while some even report an increase in sensitivity to certain types of pain with increasing age (for example, pressure pain, electrical shock, and cold pressor). These studies are summarized in Table 2 (adapted from Harkins and Warner, 1980; from Harkins and Price, 1992b).

Based on the studies summarized in Table 2, we must currently conclude that age does not have a major impact on the sensory processes subserving pain as studied to date in the laboratory in healthy, well-instructed elderly subjects (Harkins and Warner, 1980; Harkins and Price, 1992a, 1992b; Harkins et al., 1990). Nevertheless, the possibility exists that age in the later years of life does affect selective processes subserving nociception. This may relate to factors such as age-related atypical pain presentation as a symptom (for example, loss of acute, referred pain as seen in silent myocardial infarcts in the old) and the increased risk of neuropathic pain (for example, post-herpetic neuralgia) in the very old.

It is unlikely that presbyalgos should or can be defined in terms of age-related differences in need for analgesics or anaesthetics (see Table 1). The effect of age on pharmacokinetics and pharmacodynamics of analgesics and anaesthetics, fortunately, has received considerable attention. These effects seem to be dependent more on integrity of metabolic processes such as renal and hepatic functioning rather than age related developmental effects on pain. Nevertheless, there is little question that ageing in the later years of life is associated with increased risk of atypical pain presentation. This includes, as mentioned previously, increased risk of silent (painless) myocardial infarcts and presence of pain of undetermined etiology associated with degenerative disease (such as, pain associated with parkinsonism or diabetic neuropathy). In such conditions the physiological processes subserving nociception are abnormal. The manner in which ageing *per se* contributes to these abnormalities is unclear. Age may selectively influence the affective–motivation dimension of pain. This possibility has received less attention than the sensory dimension of pain.

Primary Affective Component of Pain

Table 2 presents selected characteristics of the primary affective component of pain (Price and Harkins, 1992; Harkins and Price, 1992b; Price, 1988). Possible effects of age are also listed.

Several lines of evidence suggest that age is not a major factor influencing this primary affective component of pain. Sorkin, Rudy, Hanlon, Turk and Stieg (1990) found no age effects on pain affective distress in chronic pain patients. Several studies found a consistent lack of an age effect on ratings of the primary affective response for both experimental pain (Harkins, Price, and Martelli, 1986) and clinical pain (see Figure 2).

In Figure 2 chronic pain intensity and immediate unpleasantness ratings are plotted. These are quite similar in younger and older chronic pain patients. These data are based on ratings of chronic pain by patients who met selected age and pain criteria in a multidisciplinary chronic pain diag-

Figure 2. Visual analogue scale (VAS) pain ratings

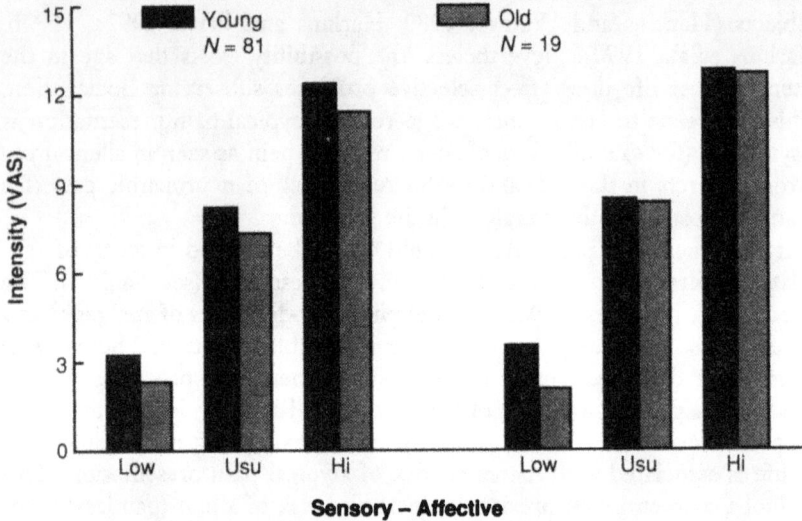

Sensory – Affective

VAS ratings of chronic pain intensity and unpleasantness in young and old patients. No statistically significant differences were observed. Pain ratings were made for pain at its lowest (low), usual (usu), and highest (hi) levels over the past week. VAS was a 150-mm line labelled 'no pain' or 'not at all unpleasant' on the extreme left and 'the most intense pain' or 'the most unpleasant pain imaginable' on the extreme right for pain intensity and pain unpleasantness, respectively. From Harkins et al. (1994; with permission).

nostic and treatment centre. The mean age for the young group (n = 81) was 35.6 years, and the mean age for the old group (n = 19) was 71.3 years. Ratings were made of pain sensory intensity at its lowest, usual, and highest levels over the past week (on a 150-millimetre visual analogue scale, VAS). Similar ratings were made for pain unpleasantness. No significant age effects were observed. This is consistent with the findings of Harkins et al. (1986) who also employed VASs to evaluate the effect of age on intensity and unpleasantness ratings of experimental pain and observed only minimal age differences in young, middle-aged, and old healthy volunteers (see also Kenshalo, 1986). Thus, it can be concluded that age in the later years of life likely does not have a dramatic effect on the primary affective component of pain.

Secondary Affective Component of Pain
As indicated in Table 2, no studies exist that have specifically evaluated the effects of age on the secondary affective component of pain. The potential

Figure 3. Interactions between different dimensions of pain

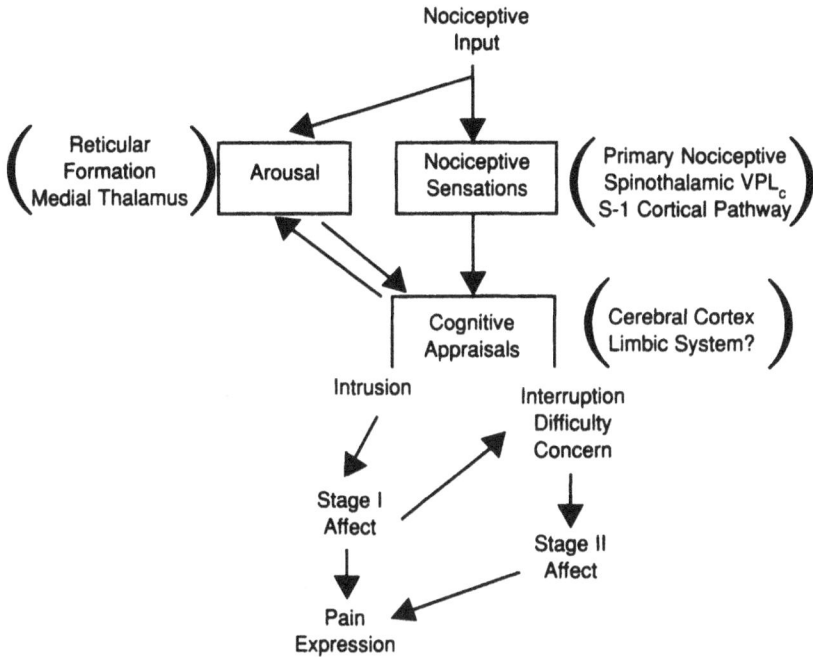

Neural structures considered to have a role in the different dimensions or stages of pain are shown in corresponding adjacent parentheses. From Price (1988); Price and Harkins (1992c); with permission.

relation of age to this component of pain is discussed below within the context of a general model of human pain based on the work of Melzack (1973) and Melzack and Wall (1965).

A MODEL FOR ASSESSMENT OF GERIATRIC PAIN

The question remains, if and how age, in the later years, influences pain. A model, shown in Figure 3, illustrating aspects of the different dimensions of pain (Melzack, 1973) may clarify these issues. This model presumes two stages of the affective–motivational dimension of pain as indicated in Table 1 (Price, 1988; Price and Harkins, 1992). The first stage is the immediate unpleasantness of pain and the second is based on cognitive processing of the longer-term implications of pain and its interactions with one's life in general.

As shown in Figure 3, nociceptive inputs trigger nociceptive sensations. Accompanied by arousal, these sensations result in cognitive appraisals, which in turn influence Stage I and Stage II affect (Harkins et al., 1986; Price and Harkins 1992; Price, 1988). The combination of these two stages of pain affect leads to the expressions of pain most frequently encountered by clinicians – pain-related suffering and pain behaviours. The information to be presented strongly supports the equivalence of nociceptive processing and primary pain-related affect (Stage I pain affect) among different age groups.

Equivalence of the Sensory–Discriminative Dimension of Pain in Young and Old

Advancing age *per se* appears to have minimal impact on either experimental or chronic pain *intensity* (see Figure 2 and Table 3). This suggests that peripheral and central neurophysiological processes subserving nociceptive sensations (see Figure 3) are little influenced by normal ageing. It must be recognized that this may not hold for all pains.

Evidence for Equivalence of Stage I Pain Affect with Ageing

Stage I pain affect, which is the primary unpleasantness of a nociceptive event (see Table 2 and Figures 2 and 3), involves the impact of nociceptive sensations on immediate feelings. This aspect of pain commands attention. It represents the intrusive aspect of nociceptive sensations on immediate activities of daily living. It involves a motivational drive to withdraw and avoid further nociceptive input combined with memory of previous similar situations. This response is related not only to the nociceptive input but also to other accompanying sensory experiences and their meanings (Price, 1988; Price and Harkins, 1992). This aspect of pain is appreciated by all as 'it feels bad.' Stage I pain affect has not been systematically evaluated in relation to age (Table 2). The available evidence from experimental studies of pain suggests no age differences in Stage I pain affect between young and old adults (Harkins et al., 1986). Emerging information on Stage I pain affect in clinical pain also suggests no age effects (see Figure 2). However, further research in this area is needed.

While nociceptive processes and primary (Stage I) pain affect may not vary dramatically with normal ageing, there is only preliminary information concerning the impact of age on secondary or Stage II pain affect.

Table 3. Summary of original tabulations of prevalence of pain lasting at least one month and present during the week immediately prior to the interview in 5,659 community-dwelling individuals. Prevalence of six selected pains, pain intensity, depression, and activities of daily living.

		Age Mean	Age SO	Neck %	Neck (N)	Back %	Back (N)	Hip %	Hip (N)	Knee %	Knee (N)	Other Joint Pain %	Other Joint Pain (N)	Stiff Joints %	Stiff Joints (N)
N	2,796	39.6	3.3	8.55	(239)	19.17	(536)	9.33	(261)	10.26	(287)	11.48	(321)	14.5	(406)
	2,863	74.7	5.5	9.71	(278)	21.34	(611)	14.98	(429)	21.31	(610)	13.66	(391)	26.1	(748)
χ^2				N.S.		4.13*		42.2***		123.7****		6.09**		117.4****	
VAS[1] Pain Intensity Young				35.18	(30.2)	31.6	(30.8)	35.7	(32.3)	32.0	(31.0)	34.7	(31.9)	37.9	(28.9)
Old				44.39	(30.6)	40.2	(32.0)	43.6	(32.0)	45.2	(31.3)	42.7	(30.5)	44.7	(29.6)
F				11.7**		21.2****		9.8**		34.3****		11.4***		14.0***	
(df)				(1,513)		(1,1129)		(1,683)		(1,878)		(1,702)		(1,1137)	
CESD[2] Young				10.8	(10.6)	10.6	(11.0)	10.2	(11.1)	10.9	(11.5)	10.67	(10.5)	12.3	(11.5)
Old				12.9	(10.8)	11.9	(9.9)	12.2	(10.1)	12.2	(10.1)	11.7	(9.4)	12.9	(10.2)
F				4.9*		4.2*		5.7*		2.62		1.85		0.74	
(df)				(1,515)		(1,1145)		(1,688)		(1,895)		(1,712)		(1,1152)	
ADL Score[3] Young				28.2	(8.7)	27.4	(7.3)	28.0	(8.2)	28.0	(8.1)	27.5	(7.7)	28.1	(7.5)
Old				35.7	(15.3)	34.6	(14.2)	36.8	(15.2)	36.0	(14.9)	35.5	(14.7)	36.3	(15.0)
F				44.1****		112.8***		75.6****		72.6****		77.6***		107.0****	
(df)				(1,515)		(1,1145)		(1,688)		(1,895)		(1,710)		(1,1152)	
Age Young				40.2	(3.1)	39.8	(3.31)	40.0	(3.1)	39.5	(3.5)	40.1	(3.45)	40.0	(3.2)
Old				75.0	(5.8)	74.6	(5.8)	75.7	(5.7)	75.1	(5.8)	74.8	(5.7)	74.7	(5.7)

Compiled from the national health and nutrition follow-up survey. From Harkins, Price, Bush, and Small, 1994.

[1] VAS = visual analogue scale.

[2] CESD = Center for Epidemiology Studies Depression Inventory (Radloff, 1977).

[3] ADL = Activities of Daily Living Inventory (Lawton, et al., 1969).

* $p < 0.05$ ** $p < 0.01$ *** $p < 0.001$ **** $p < 0.0001$

Figure 4. Visual analogue scale (VAS) secondary pain affect ratings

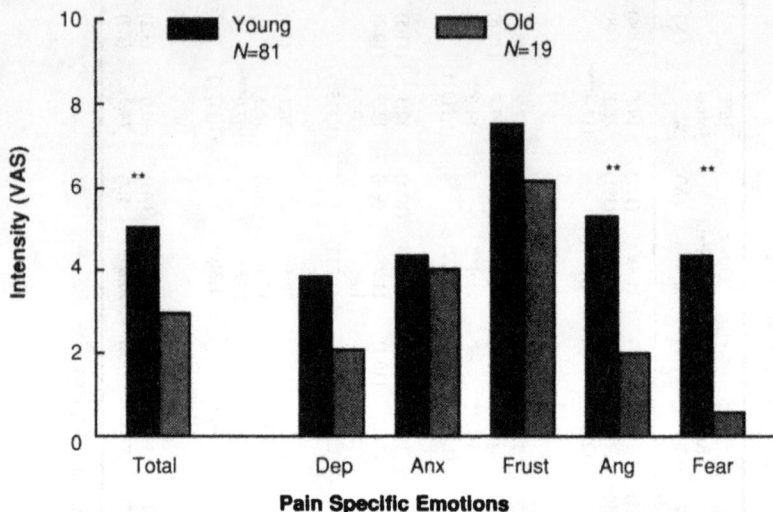

Secondary pain affect VAS ratings in young and old chronic pain patients. Data from subjects in Figure 2. (See appendix for examples of these VASs from the VCU-PAS questionnaire.)

Evidence for Age Differences in Stage II Pain Affect

Stage II pain affect depends on more elaborate cognitive appraisal than that involved in Stage I pain affect. Stage II pain affect cannot be directly evaluated in psychophysical studies of experimental pain, not only because of the artificial setting and limited meaning of experimental pain compared with clinical, recurrent or chronic pains, but also because of obvious ethical and moral concerns against producing unnecessary suffering (Price, 1988; Price and Harkins, 1992).

Figure 4 presents examples of Stage II affective responses to chronic pain measured by the Virginia Commonwealth University Pain Assessment Scale (see Appendix). The data in Figure 4 are from the same chronic pain patients whose sensory intensity and Stage I affect pain responses are shown in Figure 2. The age group differences in Stage II pain affect likely reflect age *differences, not changes,* in the meanings of pain to these two groups of individuals, most probably the result of many of the psychosocial variables mentioned earlier.

Meanings, which markedly influence Stage II affect, include perceptions of the impact of the pain on activities of daily living (interruptions), thoughts about ability to cope with the pain (tolerance of or difficulty putting up with a specific pain), and pain-related concerns for the future. These may well differ between old and young chronic pain patients. This would not necessarily reflect age differences or changes in nociceptive processes, but rather, the effect of birth cohort with its associated social history difference, life experiences with expectations of the effects of pain on daily living, and changed family and societal expectations and demands. The age group differences in Figure 4 also likely reflect the general, though erroneous assumption that pain is an expected, 'normal' consequence of growing older.

Stage II pain affect shares many properties of emotional suffering. Such suffering can be defined 'as the state of severe distress associated with events that threaten the intactness of the person' (Cassel, 1982). The confusion of clinical and chronic pain with suffering reflects the fact that disease models dominate thinking concerning pain.

Unameliorated pain-related suffering (Stage II or secondary pain affect) requires different interventions than those traditionally used for control of the sensory intensity or the primary affective components of pain. Psychological, and perhaps physiological, changes occur as a result of the prolonged presence of pain. Pain drains energy, depletes physical reserve, and lowers mood. The impact of Stage II affect on cognitive functioning has never been systematically evaluated, but in groups at risk for cognitive impairment, such as the frail elderly, it likely is considerable. Stage II pain affect is also likely a major source of psychosocial morbidity and mortality in the elderly. Its relation to drug abuse, alcoholism, and suicide in the aged needs formal evaluation.

As noted earlier, those elderly people deciding to seek a referral to the pain clinic (see Figures 2 and 4) are as likely to benefit from treatment as are young chronic pain patients (Sorkin et al., 1990). Furthermore, age does not seem to result in differences in pain coping strategies (Keefe and Williams, 1990). Elderly people attending speciality pain clinics may not, however, be representative of the general geriatric pain population. This is supported by the fact that pain is associated with considerable suffering in other elderly pain patient groups (Moss, Lawton, and Glicksman, 1991; Ferrell, Ferrell, and Osterweil, 1990; Parmelee, Katz, and Lawton, 1991; Cohen-Mansfield and Marx, 1993). Systematic evaluation of older pain patients with validated pain assessment instruments that define characteristics of nociceptive sensations, Stage I affect, Stage II affect, and pain cognitive appraisal (see Appendix), may clarify the degree of physical, social, and psychological morbidity secondary to pain in the elderly, as well as permit development of hypotheses concerning the origins of age differences in pain-related suffering and behaviour that are experimentally testable.

Coppin (1991) conducted a study of pain and its influence on ADLs in a nursing home population. The Multidimensional Pain Inventory, along with the McGill Pain Questionnaire and a visual analogue scale pain questionnaire, was employed not only to assess characteristics of the pain itself, but also to determine how pain influenced interactions with nursing staff, family, and friends. The ability to engage in and perform routine and social activities was also assessed. The results indicated that pain, depression, and limitations in day-to-day activities specifically related to pain represent a three-pronged source of suffering.

Elderly nursing home residents are an important portion of the elderly population that is considered for understanding how chronic pain contributes to and coexists with psychosocial morbidity and mortality (Parmelee, 1991; Cohen-Mansfield and Marx, 1993). A comprehensive answer to this question, with appropriate strategies for intervention, will improve the quality of life of elderly people in long-term care facilities, and may even decrease the need for more costly levels of care.

SPECIAL ISSUES RELATED TO PAIN AND PAIN TREATMENTS
IN THE ELDERLY

As noted earlier, a major problem concerning effective intervention for geriatric pain relates to a number of barriers that need to be addressed to insure adequate treatment of pain in the older individual. These barriers exist in both the assessment and treatment phases of pain management. These are presented in Table 4 along with special considerations for geriatric pain assessment and treatment.

A major barrier in assessment of pain in the old is that of 'acceptances.' There seems to be a misconception that experiencing pain is a normal part of the ageing process. This misunderstanding is often found among health care professionals, patients, and society in general. The first obstacle to overcome would be to assure the elderly pain patient that it is acceptable to admit to pain. This, of course, is the opposite of the problem encountered in the chronic pain patient with pain-related abnormal illness behaviour (Pilowsky and Spence, 1975; Harkins, Bush, Price, and Hamer, 1991).

When an individual attributes his or her pain to normal ageing, coping mechanisms may decrease the reporting of pain or the active seeking of treatment for pain (Hofland, 1992; Prohaska, Keller, Leventhal, and Leventhal, 1987). This may be more prevalent among individuals who have a tendency towards an external locus of control. There is also the possibility that an elderly patient will not report pain for fear of being viewed as a 'bad patient,' for fear that the complaint will lead to the further expense of tests, or for fear of diagnostic procedures and the treatment itself (Hofland, 1992).

Table 4. Special considerations in geriatric pain assessment and treatment

---

1. Misconceptions:
   a. Recognize that age itself does not reduce pain sensitivity.
   b. Recognize that there is no evidence that age, *per se* influences qualitative properties of pain.
   c. Recognize the importance of encouraging patient to discuss the pain.

2. Co-morbidity: Illness and symptom presentation in the elderly, particularly the frail and the 'old-old', is often characterized by multiplicity, duplicity, and chronicity.

3. Mental Status: Assess for cognitive impairment such as dementia of the Alzheimer's type, pseudo-dementia secondary to depression, and multi-infarct dementia. Referral is necessary.

4. Depression: Pain is likely a major source of depression in the elderly.

5. Activities of Daily Living (ADL): Differentiate between limitations caused by non-pain-related dysfunction and limitations in activities because their performance is painful. Pain-related dysfunction and limitation in ADLs are likely significant sources of depression in the old.

6. Medications: Assess all current and recent medications: (look in the 'Brown Bag of Pills'. Start low and go slow – and MASTER medications:
   M: Minimize number and dosages of drugs.
   A: Alternative therapies should be considered. These include recognition of the value of physical therapy.
   S: Start low and go slow.
   T: Titrate carefully.
   E: Educate patient, family, and staff that pain is not a normal part of ageing and that the frail elderly, like infants, are particularly at risk of drug interactions.
   R: Review pain and treatment strategies regularly, monitor and reassess strategies with patient and where cognitive capacity may be compromised review with patient and primary caregivers. Recognize that altered mental status may be from uncontrolled pain as well as from medications.

7. Family and Social Support Systems: Maintain these systems in the physically or mentally impaired elderly.

The next barrier in appropriate management of pain in the elderly is overcoming the misconceptions by health care professionals and the difficulties these professionals encounter in assessing the patient. Health care professionals must be aware of the factors that may inhibit a patient from reporting pain. They must take the necessary time to question and educate the patient, and they must assess other physical or behavioural indications of pain (D'Agostino, Gray, and Scanlon, 1990; Hofland, 1992).

A major challenge for health care workers in assessing pain in the elderly is with patients who have dementia, cognitive deficits, or other conditions that affect the ability to communicate. As a result of the difficulty in evaluation, these patients' pain is likely to go unrelieved (Harkins, and Price, 1992a, 1992b; Greenlee, 1991).

Once the presence of pain becomes apparent and the evaluation of the pain is complete, the next step is to devise a treatment plan. Analgesic drugs are the primary treatment for acute pain, and a major treatment for chronic pain in the elderly. Other pharmacological choices affect the symptoms associated with the pain or the condition that is creating the pain. These include antidepressants, antibiotics, anticonvulsants, neuroleptic agents, anxiolytic sedatives, and steroids (Wall, 1990).

Unfortunately, the use of medications for pain management in the elderly is not without problems. Physiological changes that occur with normal ageing and with disease processes can affect the drug's absorption, distribution, metabolism, and elimination. Absorption may be decreased or slowed in the elderly as a result of changes in the gastrointestinal system, cardiac output, muscle activity, and dehydration. Distribution may be affected by changes in body composition and cardiac output. Metabolism is generally slower in the elderly, thus prolonging the effect of the drug. Finally, elimination may be slowed as a result of decreased kidney blood flow (Greenlee, 1991). It is critical that the physician uses careful selection and monitoring of medications based on individual patients' clinical presentation, past medical history, concurrent medications, and lifestyle. Because of the complexity and problems associated with the use of drugs in the elderly, it is wise to consider alternative treatment options. Other treatment choices available for both acute and chronic pain include nerve block therapy, physiatric intervention, and psychological techniques (Wall, 1990).

Nerve block therapy involves the injection of local anaesthetics, alone or in combination with corticosteroids, into specific central or peripheral nerve sites that innervate the painful area. They may also be administered into the muscle or periosteum at the site of pain (Wall, 1990).

Physiatric intervention may include the fitting of orthoses or prostheses, occupational therapy, or physical therapy. Therapy may use strengthening or stretching exercises, education, or modalities such as heat, cold, massage, hydrotherapy, ultrasound, and electrical stimulation (Michlovitz, 1986). Transcutaneous electrical nerve stimulation (TENS) is one form of electrical stimulation that increases input through the afferent nerve fibres to modify the pain stimulus at the spinal cord and supraspinal levels of the central nervous system (Nelson and Currier, 1987).

Finally, psychological techniques are useful in the management of both acute and chronic pain. Treatment of pain has primarily concentrated on the medical areas in relation to pain control, but recently there has been more interest in the cognitive and behavioural influence on pain management. Keefe and colleagues have investigated how coping strategies are used by patients to handle their pain which in turn may affect their physical and psychological functioning. Coping strategies may include distracting oneself by other activities, ignoring the pain, reinterpreting the pain, changing activity level, praying, or hoping and using calming self-statements (Keefe et al. 1987). Based on studies of subjects with rheumatoid arthritis and osteoarthritis, it was discovered that these patients do indeed use coping strategies to help deal with their pain. Furthermore, patients who rated their ability to control and diminish the pain as high, and infrequently engaged in catastrophizing, had much lower levels of pain and psychological distress (Keefe et al. 1987, 1991). Coping strategies were correlated with adjustment to pain although the direction of the causal effect remains unknown.

Given that patients with chronic pain already engage in coping strategies to help them deal with pain, it is logical that patients be taught cognitive–behavioural techniques for pain management as a form of treatment. Stress inoculation training (SIT) is one such treatment that teaches the patient to reconceptualize the pain as a controllable event. It has been shown to have a small effect on pain intensity, but it does have a significant effect on coping ability and activity level (Puder, 1988). It is likely that individuals who tend to have an internal locus of control (LOC) will benefit from such treatment more so than those who have an external LOC. Other forms of cognitive–behavioural treatment include progressive muscle relaxation and deep breathing, attention-focusing and imagery-based pain control techniques, biofeedback, and cognitive restructuring or problem-solving skills (Middaugh, 1991; Puder, 1988).

Because of the several treatment options available for pain management, how to proceed would seem fairly straightforward. Unfortunately, the management of pain in the elderly population is complicated by the potential risks and interactions of the various treatments.

Another major barrier in pain management for the geriatric population is the referral and admission of patients into pain clinics. It is clear that the elderly are under-represented in the chronic pain settings. Figure 5 presents the age distribution for 174 consecutive chronic pain patients to a chronic pain treatment centre. The major reason for the clinic visit in these patients was musculoskeletal pain. Back pain occurred most frequently. In

Figure 5. Percentage of chronic pain patients as a function of age attending a
chronic pain diagnosis and treatment centre.

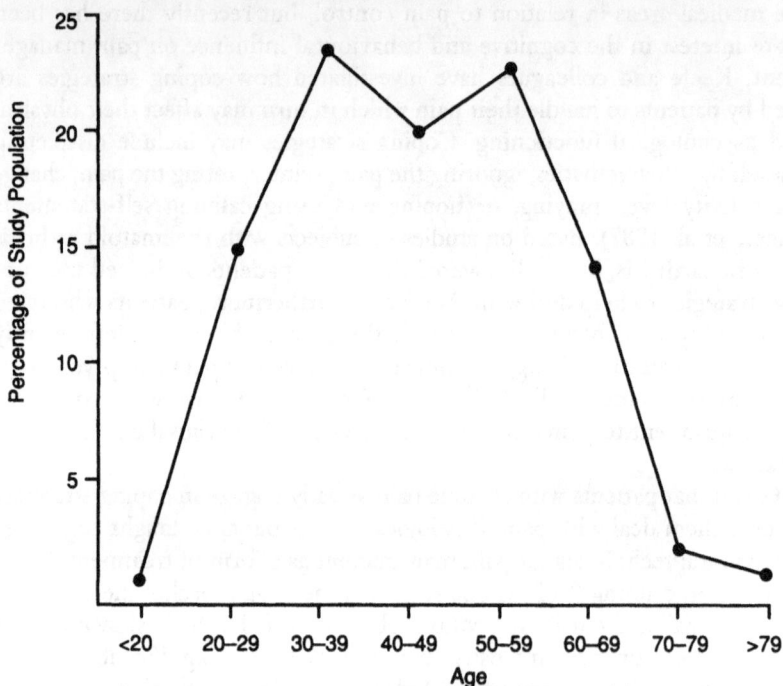

Data based on 174 consecutive patients. Reproduced from Harkins et al., 1984, with
permission.

the primary practice setting, back pain and headache do tend to decrease
with age (Harkins, 1988; Harkins et al., 1990), while degenerative problems frequently associated with pain increase (Harkins, 1988; Harkins et
al., 1990). Interestingly, it has recently been observed in the general population that persistent, recurrent, and chronic pains increase with age (Crook,
Weir, and, Tunks, 1989; Harkins, Price, Bush, and Small, 1994).

Harkins et al. (1994), in an analysis of pain data from 5,659 individuals
participating in a population-based sampling of the United States (the
NHANES Follow-up Survey), found significant increases in most forms of
musculoskeletal pain in older (n = 2,863; mean age, 74.7 years) compared
with younger (n = 2,796; mean age, 39.6 years) respondents. These findings are shown in Table 3. The older participants were more at risk for
back, hip, knee, and other joint pain compared with younger individuals. It
was also observed that older respondents had higher depression scores and

greater limitations in activities of daily living compared with younger respondents. No research has as yet systematically evaluated the relationships among age, chronic pain, depression, and limitation in activities of daily living. It is likely that impaired functioning as a result of pain is a major source of depression in the old. This has been documented, retrospectively, by psychological autopsy (Moss et al., 1991).

In previous work we have stressed that degenerative processes are likely a major source of discomfort and pain to the older individual. These results are summarized in Figure 6. Psychosocial morbidity associated with the conditions shown in Figure 6 has not been evaluated systematically in the elderly.

Age is also associated with increased risk of fracture with subsequent morbidity and mortality risks. The increase in selected fractures in a population of primary care patients (approximately 86,000 patients making over half a million patient visits to five primary care centres; Marsland, Wood, and Mayo, 1976) are illustrated in Figure 7. There has as yet been no systematic research on pain-related psychosocial morbidity associated with fractures in the later years of life. Pain consequent to fractures in this population likely is a significant contributor to decreased quality of life and unnecessary suffering in the old.

The Geriatric Pain Clinic

Multidisciplinary chronic pain rehabilitation programs are increasingly becoming the treatment of choice for chronic pain patients, although there are still the options to treat the pain from a single discipline. We have previously reported that the elderly are not frequent patients at these clinics. This finding is summarized in Figure 5, which shows the age–frequency distribution for a consecutive sample of patients attending a pain clinic. These findings seem representative of most clinics and likely reflect a referral bias on the part of primary providers, a hesitancy to accept such referrals on the part of the treating clinic, and a hesitancy to seek such referrals on the part of older patients. Mistakenly contributing clinical symptoms of pain to normal ageing, or depression, or dementia prohibits appropriate referral (Sorkin et al., 1990). Many programs are biased against accepting older patients and place a maximal age for acceptance based on assumptions that such patients will be difficult to treat and will lower the program's success rates (Middaugh et al., 1991). Another barrier for older adults to receiving treatment is the problem of limited or nonexistent reimbursement by health insurance companies (Gatz and Pearson, 1988). Pain,

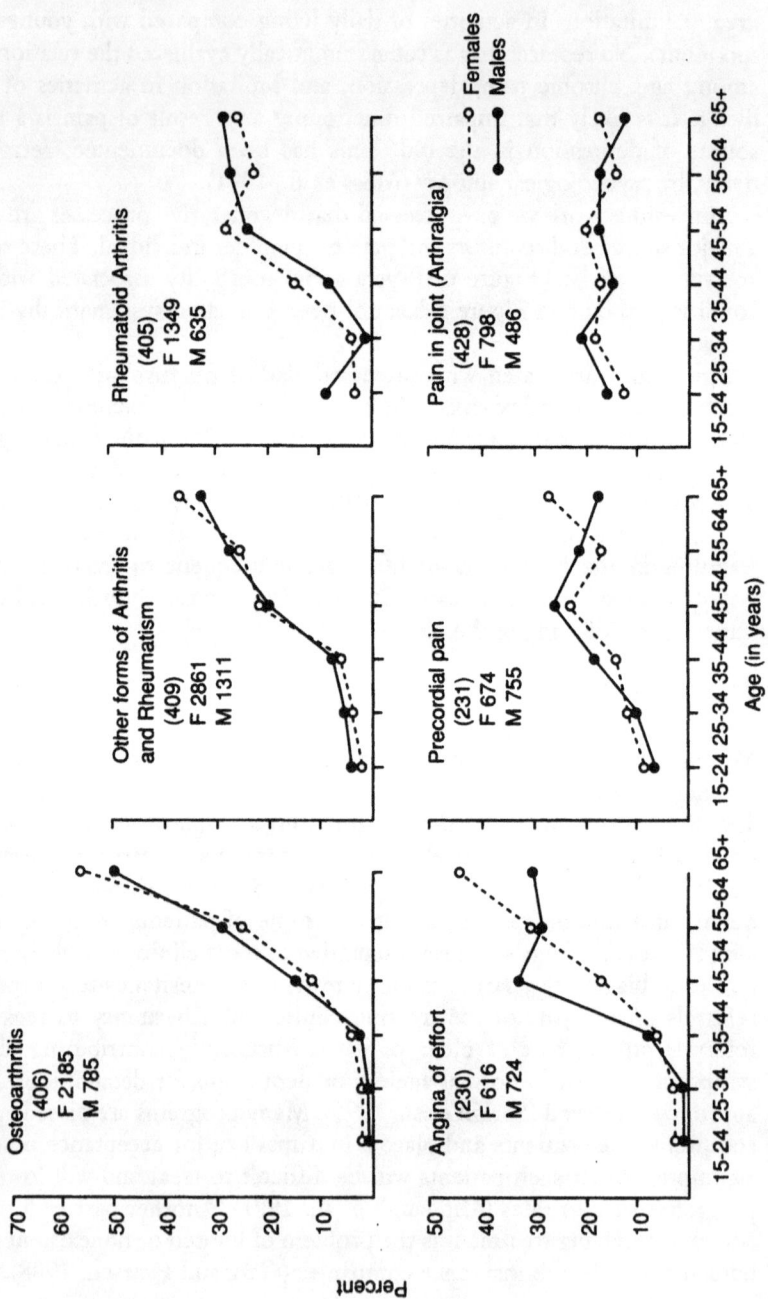

Figure 6. Frequency of primary care reasons for visit based on over half a million patient visits to primary care centres in the state of Virginia by approximately 86,000 patients.

Osteoarthritis
(406)
F 2185
M 785

Other forms of Arthritis and Rheumatism
(409)
F 2861
M 1311

Rheumatoid Arthritis
(405)
F 1349
M 635

Angina of effort
(230)
F 616
M 724

Precordial pain
(231)
F 674
M 755

Pain in joint (Arthralgia)
(428)
F 798
M 486

Females
Males

Percent

Age (in years)

15-24 25-34 35-44 45-54 55-64 65+

Original data abstracted from Marsland, 1976, as presented in Harkins et al., 1990.

Figure 7. Frequency of selected fractures by age groups in a primary care setting

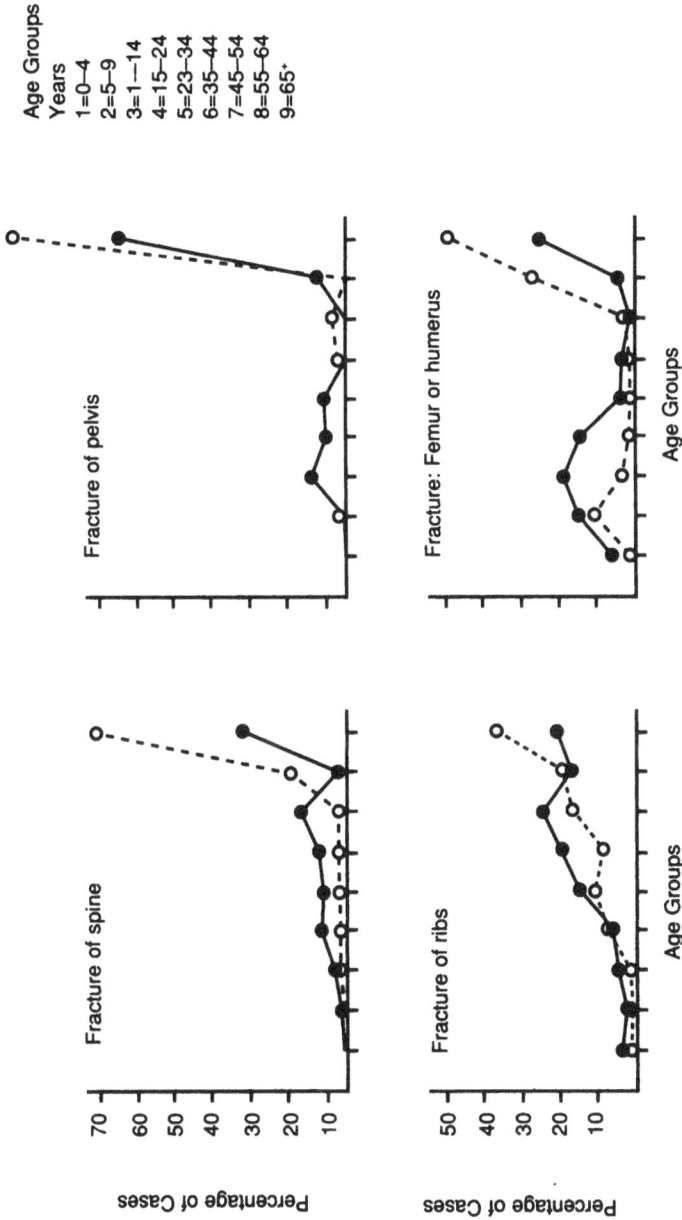

Original data abstracted from Marsland, Wood, and Mayo, 1976. From Harkins (1988).

even that of presumptive etiology, is not a 'normal' consequence of ageing in the later years of life.

As noted, diagnosis and treatment of chronic pain in the old is a major challenge because of the potential for multiple, overlapping factors contributing to pain in the elderly. Recently, attempts have been made to assess the value of a geriatric pain clinic team approach in the treatment of chronic pain in older adults. Helme and his colleagues (Helme, Katz, Neufeld, Lachal, and Corron, 1989) have established a geriatric pain clinic that accepts patients fifty-five years or older in an attempt to meet this challenge. Based on evaluation of the first hundred patients, they concluded that there is need for this type of clinic. The results indicated that chronic pain, previously unresponsive to treatment by the referring physicians, was responsive to the efforts of the geriatric pain, multidisciplinary treatment approach. Patients with musculo-skeletal pain resulting from degenerative disease, post-herpetic neuralgia, and pain of primarily psychological basis were particularly responsive to this team approach. Similar results have been reported in terms of improvement of functional status, defined in terms of increased mobility and activities of daily living in patients over sixty-five years treated in a comprehensive pain program approach (Ysla, Rosonoff, and Rosomoff, 1986). Certainly, these initial reports support the elimination of using age as a consideration in selecting a treatment.

That the elderly who attended the chronic pain clinic reported equivalent levels of pain intensity and primary pain affect and reduced pain-related suffering (secondary pain affect in Figure 4 or Stage II pain affect in the model in Figure 3) must not be over-interpreted. As demonstrated in this chapter, conditions associated with pain increase with age in primary care patients (Figures 6 and 7) and in the general population (Table 3; see Harkins et al., 1992).

In Table 3, musculoskeletal pains were shown not only to increase with age, but were reported as more painful in older compared with younger community-dwelling individuals (Harkins et al., 1992b). The impact of such pain in the general population on quality of life, risk of depression and alcoholism, limitation of activities of daily living, and psychosocial morbidity must not be underestimated. Those elderly people who are able and who choose to attend the chronic pain centre for diagnosis and treatment are most likely atypical geriatric pain patients. This may well explain the results shown in Figure 4, which likely represents elderly people with a high level of coping skills, as well as knowledge and economic resources beyond those of the majority of their age peers.

CONCLUSION

Even though the topic of pain is one that many may want to avoid, it is one that cannot be ignored. Pain, both chronic and acute, is a part of many people's lives and probably a symptom that everyone has or will experience one day. Thus far, we know that pain has physiological, affective, and cognitive dimensions. There is convincing evidence that many aspects of pain do not change as a result of normal ageing. Also, the elderly population responds well to multidisciplinary treatment. Finally, effective pain management can be complex, but there are additional intricacies in dealing with this unique group. As the geriatric population continues to grow, we as a society have a duty to dispel the myths of pain in the elderly population and to further understand how to effectively assess and treat pain. We must find how to work with and around the special issues that relate to the elderly population so that we may provide appropriate pain management. We need to find how controlled, empirical studies apply to clinical settings. The need to address these unanswered questions will become more pressing as the 'baby boomers' age. Our duty to understand pain in the aged is, however, not only determined by the sheer growth of the geriatric population, but also by the ethical demand for the humanitarian care of discomfort, pain, and suffering.

APPENDIX

The Virginia Commonwealth University Pain Inventory

There are three main parts of your pain experience that we are interested in. The first part is what the pain itself feels like, its location, duration, how intense the pain has been over the past week, and the impact of your pain on your daily activities. The second part is concerned with how bothersome and unpleasant or disturbing it is to have the painful sensation(s). Finally, the third part concerns the emotions and thoughts you have that are specifically related to your pain.

Name _____

Address _____

Age _____

Today's date _____

Date pain started _____

How long have you had this pain?   years _____ months _____

Pain Intensity and Unpleasantness of Your Pain

We are interested in knowing how intense and how bothersome (unpleasant) your pain has been to you over the past week. We are particularly interested in having you separately indicate the sensory intensity of your pain and the negative or bad feeling of unpleasantness that accompanies your pain when it occurs. People generally do not distinguish between these two aspects (intensity and unpleasantness) of pain. Pain intensity is how strong the pain feels. Pain unpleasantness is how disturbing the pain is to you. Pain unpleasantness is the bad feeling produced by pain. The distinction between these two aspects of pain might be clearer if you think of listening to music, say, from a radio. As the volume of the sound increases, you can make judgments about how loud the music is to you and you can adjust the sensory intensity of the music to the level you want to listen to. You can also make separate judgments about whether you like the music and how much you like or dislike the particular song being played at any given moment. Some people enjoy certain types of music and dislike other types no matter how loudly or softly they are played. The intensity of pain is like the loudness of the music. The unpleasantness of pain depends not only on its intensity but also on other factors that may affect you, such as the meaning of the pain to you, its impact on your activities, and many other personal factors related to the effect of pain on you.

The scales below are for measuring these two aspects of pain – pain intensity and pain unpleasantness. Some pain sensations may be equally intense and unpleasant or they may differ in their intensity and unpleasantness. Therefore, we want you to judge these two aspects of your pain independently on the scales below.

Part 1: Pain Intensity

Pain Intensity over the Past Week

Please mark the lines below with an X to indicate the relative *intensity* of your pain over the past week at its lowest, usual, highest, and current intensities. The farther to the right you place your X, the greater the intensity of your pain.

No other person can experience your pain, so there is no right or wrong answer.

Remember, enter a mark on each of the lines below, indicating your pain at its lowest, usual, and highest *instensity* over the past week.

No sensation   →   *The most intense*
                                 sensation imaginable

Lowest intensity
of pain   _____

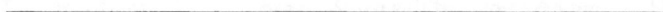

Usual intensity
of pain _____

Highest intensity
of pain _____

Current intensity
of pain _____

Part 2: Pain Unpleasantness

Your Pain Unpleasantness over the Past Week

Please mark the lines below with an X to indicate the relative *unpleasantness* of your
pain over the past week at its lowest, usual, and highest levels. The farther to the
right you place your X, the greater the *unpleasantness* of your pain.
    No other person can experience your pain, so there is no right or wrong answer.
    Remember, enter a mark on each of the lines below, indicating your pain at its
lowest, usual, and highet *unplesantness* over the past week.

	Not at all *unplesant or* *bothersome*	*The most unpleasant* *or bothersome* *imaginable*

Lowest level of
pain unpleasantness _____

Usual level of
pain unpleasantness _____

Highest level of
pain unpleasantness _____

Current level of
pain unpleasantness _____

Part 3

It is not unusual to perceive negative emotions regarding pain. We want to know
the kinds of feelings that accompany or are associated with your pain, and we also
want to know how intense they are.
    Just as you marked the level of sensory pain intensity and of your pain unpleas-

antness, we want you to mark with an X the intensity of specific negative emotions associated with your pain over the past week.

Simply mark the extent of each feeling, as appropriate, on the lines below.

	None (0%)	*The most intense or severe imaginable* (100%)
1. Depression		
2. Anxiety		
3. Frustration		
4. Anger		
5. Fear		

For each of the following, mark an X along the scale supplied to indicate the extent of your experience or feeling. Remember, the farther to the right, the greater the extent.

How much does your pain prevent you from doing what you want to do?

No interference   Complete interference

How difficult is it to endure the pain over time?

Not at all difficult   Extremely difficult

How concerned are you about future harm or impaired health?

Not at all concerned   Most concerned

In general, how likely do you think it is that your pain can be removed or cured?

Impossible   Certain

How likely do you think it is that this clinic will remove your pain?

Impossible   Certain

In general, to what extent do you feel you have control over your own health?

No control   Complete control

In general, to what extent can you reduce the intensity of your pain?

0%	100%

REFERENCES

Birren, J.E., Shapiro, H.B., & Miller, J.H. (1950). The effect of salicylate upon pain sensitivity. *Journal of Pharmacological and Experimental Therapy, 100*, 67–71.

Bonica, J.J. (1990). *The Management of Pain* (2nd ed.). Philadelphia: Lea & Febiger.

Chapman, W.P., & Jones, C.M. (1944). Variations in cutaneous and visceral pain sensitivity in normal subjects. *Journal of Clinical Investigation, 23*, 81–91.

Clark, W.C. & Mehl, L., (1971). Thermal pain: A sensory decision theory analysis of the effect of age and sex on various response criteria, and 50 per cent pain threshold. *Journal of Abnormal Psychology, 78*, 202–12.

Cohen-Mansfield, J., & Marx, M.S. (1993). Pain and depression in the nursing home: corroborating results. *Journal of Gerontology, 48*, 96–7.

Collins, G., and Stone, L.A. (1966). Pain sensitivity, age, and activity level in chronic schizophrenics and in normals. *British Journal of Psychiatry, 112*, 33–5.

Crisson, J.E., & Keefe, F.J. (1988). The relationship of locus of control to pain coping strategies and psychological distress in chronic pain patients. *Pain, 35*, 147–54.

Critchley, M. (1931). The neurology of old age. *Lancet*, vol. 1, *225*, 1221–30.

Crook, J., Weir, R., & Tunks, E. (1989). An epidemiological follow-up survey of persistent pain sufferers in a group family practice and specialty pain clinic. *Pain, 36*, 49–61.

D'Agostino, N.S., Gray, G., & Scanlon, C. (1990). Cancer in the older adult: Understanding age-related changes. *Journal of Gerontological Nursing, 16*, 12–15.

Elliott, T.R., & Harkins, S.W. (1991). Psychosocial concomitants of persistent pain among persons with spinal cord injuries. *NeuroRehabilitation, 1*, 7–19.

Elliott, T., & Harkins, S.W. (1992). Emotional distress and the perceived interference of menstruation. *Journal of Psychopathology and Behavioral Assessment, 14*, 293–306.

Ferrell, B.A., Ferrell, B.R., & Osterweil, D. (1990). Pain in the nursing home. *Journal of the American Geriatrics Society, 38*, 409–14.

Fozard, J.L. (1990). Vision and hearing in aging. In: J.E. Birren & K. Warner Schaie (Eds.), *Handbook of the Psychology of Aging*, (3rd ed.). New York: Academic Press, 150–70.

France, R.D. (1989). Psychiatric aspects of pain. *Clinical Journal of Pain, 5*, S35–S42.

Fries, J.F. (1980). Aging, natural death, and the compression of morbidity. *New England Journal of Medicine, 300*, 130–5.

Fries, J.F., Green, L.W., & Levine, S. (1989). Health promotion and the compression of morbidity. *Lancet, 4*, 481–3.

Gatz, M., & Pearson, C.G. (1988). Ageism revised and the provision of psychological services. *American Psychologist, 43*, 184–8.

Gil, K.M., Keefe, F.J., Crisson, J.E., & Van Dalfsen, P.J. (1987). Social support and pain behavior. *Pain, 29*, 209–17.

Greenlee, K.K. (1991). Pain and analgesia: Considerations for the elderly in critical care. *AACN Clinical Issues, 2*, 720–8.

Hardy, J.D., Wolff, H.G., & Goodell, H. (1943). The pain threshold in man. *American Journal of Psychiatry, 99*, 744–51.

Harkins, S.W. (1988). Pain in the elderly. In: R. Dubner, F.G. Gebhart, & M.R. Bond (Eds.), *Proceedings of the 5th World Congress on Pain*, Elsevier Science Publisher B.V. (Biomedical Divison), 355–7.

Harkins, S.W., Bush, F.M., Price, D.D., & Hamer, R.M. (1991) Symptom report in orofacial pain patients: Relation to chronic pain, experimental pain, illness behavior, and personality. *Clinical Journal of Pain*, 7: 102–13.

Harkins, S. W., & Chapman, C.R. (1976). Detection and decision factors in pain perception in young and elderly men. *Pain, 2*, 253–64.

Harkins, S.W., & Chapman, C.R. (1977a). The perception of induced dental pain in young and elderly women. *Journal of Gerontology, 32*, 428–35.

Harkins, S.W., & Chapman, C.R. (1977b). Age and sex differences in pain perception. In: B. Anderson, & B. Matthews (Eds.), *Pain in the Trigeminal Region*. Amsterdam: Elsevier/ North-Holland, 435–41.

Harkins, S.W., Kwentus, J., & Price, D.D. (1984). Pain and the elderly. In: C. Benedetti, C.R. Chapman, & G. Morieca (Eds.), *Advances in Pain Research and Therapy*. New York: Raven Press, vol. 7, 103–212.

Harkins, S.W., Kwentus, J., & Price, D. D. (1990). Pain and suffering in the elderly. In: J.J. Bonica (Ed.), *Management of Pain*, (2nd ed.). Philadelphia: Lea & Febiger, 552–9.

Harkins, S.W., & Price, D.D. (1992a). Are there special needs for pain assessment in the elderly? *Bulletin of American Pain Society,3*, 5–6.

Harkins, S.W., & Price, D.D. (1992b) Turk Book. Assessment of pain in the elderly. In: D.C. Turk, & R. Melzack, *Handbook of pain assessment*. New York: Gilford Press 315–31.

Harkins, S.W., Price, D.D., & Braith, J. (1989). Effects of extraversion and neuroticism on experimental pain, clinical pain, and illness behavior. *Pain, 36*, 209–18.

Harkins, S.W., Price, D.D., Bush, F.M., & Small, R. (1994). Geriatric pain. In:

P.D. Wall , & R. Melzack, *Textbook of Pain*. Edinburgh: Churchill Livingston. 769–86.

Harkins, S.W., Price, D.D., & Martelli, M. (1986). Effects of age on pain perception: Thermonociception. *Journal of Gerontology, 41*, 58–63.

Harkins, S.W., & Warner, M.H. (1980). Age and pain. In: C. Eisdorfer (Ed.), *Annual Review of Gerontology and Geriatrics*, New York: Springer–Verlag, vol. 1, 121–31.

Helme, R.D., Katz, B., Neufeld, S., Lachal, J., & Corron, H.T. (1989). The establishment of a geriatric pain clinic: A preliminary report of the first 100 patients. *Australian Journal on Ageing, 8*, 27–30.

Hofland, S.L. (1992). Elder beliefs: Blocks to pain management. *Journal of Gerontological Nursing, 18*, 19–24.

Keefe, F.J., Caldwell, D.S., Martinez, S., Nunley, J., Beckham, J., & Williams, D.A. (1991). Analyzing pain in rheumatoid arthritis patients: Pain coping strategies in patients who have had knee replacement surgery. *Pain, 46*, 153–60.

Keefe, F.J., Caldwell, D.S., Queen, K.T., Gil, K.M., Martinez, S., & Crisson, J.E. (1987). Pain coping strategies in osteoarthritis patients. *Journal of Consulting and Clinical Psychology, 55*, 208–12.

Keefe, F.J., & Williams, D.A. (1990). A comparison of coping strategies in chronic pain patients in different age groups. *Journal of Gerontology, 45*, 161–5.

Kenshalo, D.R., Sr (1986). Somesthetic sensitivity in young and elderly humans. *Journal of Gerontology, 41*, 732–42.

Lawton, M.P., & Brody, E.M. (1969). Assessment of older people: Self-maintaining and instrumental activities of daily living. *Gerontologist, 9*, 179–86.

Marsland, D.W., Wood, M., & Mayo, F. (1976). *Content of Family Practice: A Statewide Study in Virginia with Its Clinical, Educational, and Research Implications.* New York: Appleton-Century-Crofts.

Melding, P.S. (1991). Is there such a thing as geriatric pain? *Pain, 46*, 119–21.

Melzack, R. (1973). *The Puzzle of Pain*, New York: Basic Books.

Melzack, R., & Wall, P.O. (1965). Pain mechanisms: A new theory. *Science, 150*, 971–9.

Michlovitz, S.L. (1986). *Thermal Agents in Rehabilitation*. Philadelphia: Davis.

Middaugh, S.J., Woods, S.E., Kee, W.G., Harden, N., & Peters, J.R. (1991). Biofeedback-assisted relaxation training for the aging chronic pain patient. *Biofeedback and Self-regulation, 16*, 361–77.

Moss, M.S., Lawton, M.P., & Glicksman, A. (1991). The role of pain in the last year of life of older persons. *Journal of Gerontology, 46*, 51–7.

Mumford, J.M. (1965). Pain perception, threshold and adaptation of normal human teeth. *Archives of Oral Biology, 10*, 957–68.

Mumford, J.M. (1968). Pain perception in man on electrically stimulating the teeth. In: A. Soulairac, J. Cahn, & J. Charpentier (Eds.), *Pain*. London: Academic Press, 224–9.

Nelson, R.M., & Currier, D.P. (1987). *Clinical Electrotherapy*. Norwalk, CN: Appleton-Century-Crofts.

Olsho, L.W., Harkins, S.W., & Lenhardt, M.L. (1985). Aging and the auditory system. In: J.E. Bitten & K.W. Schzie (Eds.), *Handbook of the Psychology of Aging*. New York: Van Nostrand Reinhold, 332–77.

Parmelee, P.A., Katz, I.R., Lanton, M.P. (1991). The realtion of pain to depression among institutionalized aged. *Journal of Gerontology, 46,* 15–21.

Pilowsky, I. & Spence, N.D. (1975). Patterns of illness behavior in patients with intractable pain. *Journal of Psychosomatic Research, 19,* 187–279.

Price, D.D. (1988) *Psychological and Nerval Mechanisms of Pain*. New York: Raven Press.

Price, D.D., & Harkins, S.W. (1992). The affective-motivational dimension of pain. *APS Journal, 1.*

Procacci, P., Bozza, G., Buzzelli, G., & Della Corte, M. (1970). The cutaneous pricking pain threshold in old age. *Gerontology Clinics, 12,* 213–18.

Procacci, P., Della Corte, M., Zoppi, M., Romano, S., Maresca, M., & Voegelin, M. (1974). Pain threshold measurement in man. In J.J. Bonica, P. Procacci, & C. Pagoni (Eds.), *Recent Advances on Pain: Pathophysiology and Clinical Aspects*. Springfield, Il: Charles C. Thomas, 105–47.

Prohaska, T.R., Keller, M.L., Leventhal, E.A., & Leventhal, H. (1987). Impact of symptoms and aging attribution on emotions and coping. *Health Psychology, 6,* 495–514.

Puder, R.S. (1988). Age analysis of cognitive-behavioral group therapy for chronic pain outpatients. *Psychology and Aging, 3,* 204–7.

Radloff, L.S. (1977). The CES-D Scale: A self-report depression scale for research in the general population. *Applied Psychology Measurement, 1,* 385–401.

Saxon, S.V. (1991). *Pain Management Techniques for Older Adults*. Springfield, Il: Charles C. Thomas.

Schumacher, G.A., Goodell, H., Hardy, J.D., & Wolff, H.G. (1940). Uniformity of the pain threshold in man. *Science, 92,* 110–112.

Sherman E.D., & Robillard, E. (1964a). Sensitivity to pain in relationship to age. In: P.F. Hansen (Ed.), *Age with a Future: Proceedings of the 6th International Congress of Gerontology, Copenhagen, 1963*. Philadelphia: Davis, 325–33.

Sherman, E.D., & Robillard, E. (1964b). Sensitivity to pain in the aged. *Canadian Medical Association Journal, 83,* 944–7.

Skevington, S.M. (1983). Chronic pain and depression: Universal or personal helplessness? *Pain, 15,* 309–17.

Sorkin, B.A., Rudy, T.E., Hanlon, R.B., Turk, D.C., & Stieg, R.L. (1990). Chronic pain in old and young patients: Differences appear less important than similarities. *Journal of Gerontology*, *45*, 64–8.

Tucker, M.A., Andrew, M.F., Ogle, S.J., Davidson, J.G. (1989). Age associated change in pain threshold measured by transcutaneous neuronal electrical stimulation. *Age and Aging*, *18*, 241–6.

Wall, R.T. (1990). Use of analgesics in the elderly. *Clinical Pharmacology*, *6*, 345–7.

Wallston, B.S., Alagna, S.W., Devellis, B.M., & Devellis, R.F. (1983). Social support and physical health. *Health Psychology*, *2*, 367–91.

Walsh, N.E., Schoenfeld, L., Ramamurthy, S., & Hoffman, J. (1989). Normative model for cold pressor test. *American Journal of Physical Medical Rehabilation*, *68*, 6–11.

Wegman, M.E. (1990). Annual summary of vital statistics 1989. *Pediatrics*, *86*, 835–47.

Williams, A.K., & Schulz, R. (1988). Association of pain and physical dependency with depression in physically ill middle-aged and elderly persons. *Physical Therapy*, *68*, 1226–30.

Woodrow, K.M., Friedman, G.D., Siegelaub, A.B., & Collen, M.F. (1972). Pain tolerance: Differences according to age, sex, and race. *Psychosomatic Medicine*, *34*, 548–56.

8

The Combined Forces of Traditional Chinese and Western Medicine to Treat Pain in the Elderly

STEVEN K.H. AUNG

The role of the pain clinic in treating chronic pain as it strikes or afflicts the elderly individual is, above all, a 'unitary whole experience' (Roy, Bellissimo, and Tunks, 1990, p. 5). This chapter focuses on elderly patients, each of them experiencing the unitary whole experience of chronic pain, and nearly all of them referred to my ten-year-old Traditional Chinese Medicine (TCM) private practice pain clinic in downtown Edmonton, Alberta, by physicians from across Western Canada. These physicians had searched for and failed to find in these instances 'a determinate organic origin of persistent pain ... How frustrating it is for the physician to be confronted by a complaining patient whose pain remains' (Violon, 1990, p. 31). How frustrating, as well, for the patient who may end up consulting 'charlatans and healers' (Violon, 1990, p. 35). As a TCM practitioner as well as a Western family and geriatrics physician, I consider myself a healer in the widest sense of the term. Much of what I practice in my clinic, involving approximately forty patients a day, is acupuncture, which is only one TCM therapy. The efficacy of acupuncture is controversial, but I have found that acupuncture helps relieve elderly patients of their chronic pain.

This chapter is organized as follows. First, the chronic pain complaints of the elderly are reviewed, and then the role of the biomedical pain centre in addressing these complaints is considered. Then, relevant TCM concepts and therapies are outlined, the acupuncture controversy is discussed, and a concise case study of my own TCM pain clinic is presented. While the chapter is oriented towards synthesizing the relevant literature, the case study is based largely on my own knowledge and experience. The perspective informing this chapter relates to both medical pluralism and multicultural health care: Leslie (1980) argues that modern biomedicine has defined itself as dominant, ignoring or derogating the other legitimate medical systems in the world; Masi (1988) argues that Canadian physicians, working in an inherently multicultural society, should adopt a more open, culturally sensitive attitude to health care. These arguments imply the legitimacy of practising TCM in Canada, a legitimacy more precisely indicated by the biomedical referral of patients to this 'other' system.

PAIN CLINICS AND THE ELDERLY

In bringing the elderly into the pain clinic picture, it may be stated, first of all, that directories such as Oryx Press (1989) provide little evidence of the existence of geriatrics-oriented pain clinics or geriatrics-oriented programs within these clinics. Second, in what is perhaps the only pain clinic textbook as such (Diamond and Coniam, 1991) the elderly are not mentioned. Third, the elderly manifest a 'central tendency' of absence rather than presence in the multidisciplinary pain clinics (MPCs) referred to in this section of the chapter, with the possible exception of the Montefiore Hospital and Medical Centre, which has reported that 43 per cent of its first 200 patients were over sixty years old (Kepes, 1981). The absence of the elderly in pain clinics is noted by Harkins, Kwentus, and Price (1984, p. 113): 'It would appear the elderly are under-represented as a group in the chronic pain clinic setting. Only a small percentage of patients with chronic low back pain and other painful chronic musculoskeletal disorders (usually managed by family physicians, orthopaedists, and psychiatrists) and only about 10 to 25 per cent of those with chronic cancer pain (who are cared for by oncologists or family physicians) are referred to pain control clinics. No formal demographic data exist to support the possible under-utilization of pain clinics by the elderly. Considering that the elderly under-utilize health care opportunities in general, it would not be surprising to find them under-represented in pain clinics.'

While Jamison, Rock, and Parris (1988) and Turk (1990) found no differences related to age in their studies of meaningful subgroups of patients, it is likely that the elderly were under-represented in their samples. Aronoff and Wagner (1988) cite a Boston Pain Centre study finding to the effect that only age could 'predict' outcome (it was negatively correlated with improvement). Vasudevan (1988), reviewing the relevant literature, found that unsuccessful pain clinic patients tended, among other things, to be older. The rationale behind the pediatric pain management program at the University of Washington MPC, according to Tyler, Smith, Womack, and Pomietto (1989, p. 161), is that 'children respond differently than adults to all sorts of stimuli, including pain, and many of the differences are age

Table 1. Symptoms treated and therapies provided by over 70% of 477 American and
Canadian pain facilities, April 1988 to February 1989[a]

Symptom modalities	Therapy modalities
Myofascial syndromes (93%)	Physical therapy (87%)
Headache (87%)	Transcutaneous stimulation (83%)
Back pain – low (87%)	Relaxation training (82%)
Back pain – other (86%)	Drug therapies (78%)
Causalgic syndromes (85%)	Comprehensive pain management (78%)
Neuralgias (84%)	Biofeedback (78%)
Orofacial pain (76%)	Psychotherapy (75%)
Phantom limb pain (75%)	Nerve blocks (74%)
Arthritis (71%)	

[a] Compiled from Oryx Press (1989, pp. 140–201)

related.' There is no comparable program for the elderly at this MPC,
although a similar rationale could be provided with respect to the elderly
(see Table 1 for an overview of problems and their treatment at pain
clinics).

There appear to be two general explanations for the relative absence of
the elderly in pain clinics: First, drawing upon Kotarba (1981), there is less
demand from government agencies and insurance companies for successful
treatment of the elderly, because the elderly are not part of the work force
and are not receiving relatively generous compensation or insurance benefits; second, Melding (1991) suggests that covert 'ageism' pervades the
biomedical profession.

Moya and Mayne (1986) provide a rare, but brief, account of the Mount
Sinai Medical Centre in Miami, Florida, which has a geriatrics-oriented
MPC. Established in 1972, it is a private-practice out-patient facility located in the Department of Anesthesiology. It has a medical director, two
full-time physicians, and several therapists, including a social worker, hyp-
notist, and acupuncturist. This MPC receives referrals from all over the
world, and in 1982 conducted about 3,000 consultations/treatments, the
patients averaging seventy years of age. The most common problems seen
were chronic back pain (38 per cent), herpetic neuralgia (13 per cent),
skeletal/myofascial pain (13 per cent), headaches (9 per cent), and cancer
pain (5 per cent). The chronic pain syndromes found most amenable to
therapy are back pain, herpetic neuralgia, headaches, pancreatic cancer,
and causalgia. The problems found least amenable to therapy were tha-
lamic pain syndrome, peripheral neuritis, and phantom limb pain. The

most commonly used therapeutic modalities were trigger point blocks (20 per cent), epidural or spinal steroids (18 per cent), medical hypnosis (17 per cent), herpetic neuralgia blocks (9 per cent), acupuncture (9 per cent), TENS (6 per cent), and psychosocial counselling, used in almost all patients (Moya and Mayne, 1986, p. 26).

Finally, two recent – and rare – comparative studies involving small samples of the elderly pain clinic population are noteworthy. Middaugh, Levin, Kee, Barchiesi, and Roberts (1988) compared elderly and younger patients (average ages of 62.4 and 38.5, and age ranges from fifty-five to seventy-eight and twenty-nine to forty-eight, respectively) at the Medical University of South Carolina MPC and found that the former, although initially more dysfunctional, benefited more from the treatments provided. Roy, Thomas, and Berger (1990) compared patients in an urban British pain clinic and members of a Canadian urban social and recreational club, with both groups averaging just over seventy-four years of age. They found that the former were more socially isolated and experienced more chronic pain.

The actual role of pain clinics in treating elderly patients, then, is a circumscribed one. However, pain clinics do have a potential role, and a model of this is presented in Table 2. The model assumes the existence of geriatric chronic pain, as a biological, psychological, and social – or biopsychosocial – problem, and it assumes the existence of a meaningful category of chronic pain sufferers aged sixty-five and older. The model is that of an MPC organized around, designed for, and enacted in partnership with elderly patients, their families, and community volunteers. Patients are not refused admission because they are too frail or stressed, but are admitted to appropriate treatment subgroups, encompassing the dysfunctional (disabled, older elderly), adaptive copers (active, younger elderly), the distressed (potentially less active, 'middle-aged' elderly). The model emphasizes careful diagnosis, appropriate use of medication, multimodal treatment (particularly non-pharmacological, active modalities), patient awareness, patient involvement and self-rehabilitation, curing, and coping.

TCM, ACUPUNCTURE, AND WESTERN BIOMEDICINE

Having peaked as a medical system from the seventh to fourteenth centuries, TCM began to decline, and by the end of the 1920s it had been driven underground. In 1929, for example, legislation passed by the Kuomintang government in China made TCM illegal. However, after the founding of

Table 2. Geriatric pain clinic: Potential biopsychosocial, multimodal model centring around structure, process, and outcome [a]

Variables	Possible Relevant Indicators
Structural	– University, hospital, or community health/recreational centre custom-designed for elderly patients
	– Physicians and consultants (including geriatrics specialists); geriatrics-oriented nurses, physical therapists, psychological and recreational counsellors, social workers, and family and community volunteers
Processual	– Intensive biopsychosocial diagnosis and assessment
	– Patients assigned on basis of condition to (1) 'dysfunctional,' (2) 'distressed,' and (3) 'adaptive' subgroups
	– General (multimodal) treatment for each subgroup; various medical and 'non-medical' treatments for individuals
	– Emphasis on awareness, learning, and self-rehabilitation
Outcome	– Reduced and/or more appropriate medication intake
	– Cure of pathophysiological chronic pain condition or decrease in chronic pain level
	– Increased physical/recreational activity
	– Increased ability to cope with major life stressors
	– Increased recreational social activity

[a] Synthesis of Portenoy and Farkash (1988) and references cited in the text, notably Roy, Bellissimo, and Tunks (1990), Walker et al. (1990), Melding (1991), and Turk (1991)

the People's Republic of China in 1949 TCM was revitalized and officially integrated with Western biomedicine (Pei, 1983). The People's Republic remained closed to the West until the American diplomatic opening in the early 1970s. One of the first biomedical researchers to visit China, John Bonica (1974), writing in the *Journal of the American Medical Association*, expressed concern about the efficacy of acupuncture (which was receiving considerable publicity in the West), calling for controlled clinical trials. The integration of TCM into national and subnational Western medical systems depends largely on whether these systems are 'monopolistic' or 'tolerant' (Stepan, 1983). Monopolistic systems, exemplified by France, attempt to restrict all healing ('medical') practices, including acupuncture, to physicians, while tolerant systems, including the United States, Britain, and Canada, allow some healing ('non-medical') practices to be carried out by non-physicians.

Acupuncture in Context

TCM had 'as early as the second century BC ... formed its special character, combining systematic theories with rich practical experience' (Jinfeng,

1988, p. 521). *The Yellow Emperor's Sacred Canon of Medicine*, dating from the Han Dynasty (206 BC to AD 221), contains the systematic theoretical doctrine of *yin* and *yang* as well as a vast amount of information on acupuncture and other therapies.

The theoretical foundations of TCM are aptly summarized by Xinnong (1987, p. 12) as follows: 'The opposition of yin and yang is mainly reflected in their ability to struggle with, and thus control each other. For instance, warmth and heat (yang) may dispel cold, while coolness and cold (yin) may lower a high temperature. The yin or yang aspect within any phenomenon will restrict the other through opposition. Under normal conditions in the human body, therefore, a relative physiological balance is maintained through the mutual opposition of yin and yang. If for any reason this mutual opposition results in an excess or deficiency of yin or yang, the relative physiological balance of the body will be destroyed, and disease will arise.'

While TCM may appear 'unscientific' from a Western point of view, it may more properly be said to embody a qualitative scientific approach. Chinese medicine at all times has employed the inductive and synthetic approach, directly yielding statements on functions. 'If we attempt to define similar functions with reference to space, the criterion is not their quite illusive respective dimensions but ... their relative direction. Now a statement on relative direction is a qualitative statement. Because of this, Chinese medicine ... must have constant recourse to *standards of value* ... such as yin and yang ... as well as their numerous technical derivations (Porkert, 1976, p. 63, original emphasis).

TCM diagnostic techniques encompass inquiry (regarding the patient's dietary habits, medication intake, personal/family situation, and so on), inspection of the patient's body (notably the tongue, which indicates imbalance in the internal organs), taking of the pulse (in each hand there are three superficial pulses, indicating the condition of hollow organs such as the stomach, and three deep pulses, indicating the condition of solid organs such as the spleen), and palpation of acupoints (notably the twelve 'alarm' points, which are associated with the major internal organs and reflect pathophysiological changes in these organs).

Acupuncture entails the 'needling' of specific points on the body related to the meridians and their collateral, the object being to stimulate the 'arrival' of *qi* ('vital energy'), thereby helping to maintain or restore an individual's health and to relieve any pain associated with poor health. The stone or bone needles used in ancient times have been replaced by sterile, disposable, stainless steel needles, which are inserted into the patient to the right depth, manipulated, and then retained, with the precise angle, depth, degree of manipulation, and time of retention being 'qualities' of the therapeutic relationship between the acupuncturist and patient. The arrival of *qi* is indicated by the acupuncturist feeling tension through the needle (it feels like a fish biting a hook) and the patient feeling soreness, numbness, and/or heaviness around the needle.

Acupoints – and there are 361 classical points – may be local, remote, or symptomatic. Thus, a point near the eye may be stimulated to treat an eye condition, a stomach channel point on the lower leg stimulated to treat stomach ache, and a large intestine channel point stimulated to treat fever because of this point's symptomatic, fever-reducing function (Jirui and Wang, 1988, pp. 3–17; see World Health Organization, 1991, for the standardized acupoint nomenclature). Combinations of points are generally used. Electro-acupuncture, which entails the application of electric current to the acupoints through the retained needles, is frequently used to treat intense chronic pain.

Taken together, TCM diagnosis and acupuncture therapy constitute an intensive, holistic process that attempts to address both 'disease' and 'illness.' Disease implies a biomedically defined clinical entity – but illness implies the 'lived experience of illness in the practical world of everyday life. Personal, interactional, and cultural norms guide this lived experience' (Kleinman, 1986, p. 144).

Acupuncture remains controversial. The National Council Against Health Fraud (1991), for example, argues that two decades of scientific research have failed to demonstrate the efficacy of acupuncture, while others (notably Patel, 1987; Guillaume, 1991) suggest that its efficacy cannot be demonstrated in strictly biomedical terms, because the primary aim of acupuncture is to help maintain an individual's health, the energy of *qi* is difficult for researchers to conceptualize or measure, the precise combination of acupoints utilized by the acupuncturist varies with each patient, and the 'double blind' research design is difficult to attain. Moreover, two recent meta-analyses of the literature on acupuncture and chronic pain have arrived at conflicting results: Patel, Gutzwiller, Paccaud, and Marazzi (1989, p. 905), synthesizing the data from fourteen controlled studies, found that acupuncture was efficacious 'significantly more often than chance alone would allow'; Riet, Kleijnen, and Knipschild (1990), assessing fifty-one controlled studies on the basis of their methodologies, found that they were not of sufficiently high quality to prove the efficacy of acupuncture. Yet acupuncture has attained a degree of legitimacy in the biomedical system, largely within the context of chronic pain management. Thus, inspecting the directory of 477 Canadian and American pain clinics referred to earlier in this chapter indicates that 139 of the pain clinics – 41 per cent university-based and 27 per cent hospital-based – provided acupuncture therapy. Furthermore, the TENS therapy provided by over 80 per cent of the 477 centres (see again Table 1) historically derives from electro-acupuncture, and TENS has been effectively applied at TCM acupoints (Mannheimer & Lampe, 1984; Cheng & Pomeranz, 1987). At the international level, the World Health Organization has recognized the importance of alternative therapies, suggesting, for example, that acupuncture may be appropriate in treating disorders involving the upper respiratory tract, respiratory system, eyes, mouth, intestinal tract, neurological system, and musculoskeletal system (Bannerman, 1979, p. 27).

It must be noted that some of the apparent clinical efficacy of both TENS and acupuncture is explained by the biomedical gate control theory of pain (see Raj, 1986b), and at least one controlled study (Kreitler, Kreitler, and Carasso, 1987) suggests that chronic pain patients having beliefs oriented towards the relief of pain are likely to benefit from acupuncture.

AN INTEGRATED APPROACH

In my own private-practice clinic in Edmonton acupuncture is utilized for treating both non-painful and painful conditions, with 46 per cent of my patients suffering from chronic benign pain and 9 per cent cancer pain. My practice, therefore, may be termed a private-practice, modality-oriented pain clinic. It is also a geriatric clinic, because over half my patients are aged sixty-five or older. Virtually all of these elderly patients have experienced pain for two years or longer, which is why they were referred to my clinic. The complaints of these patients centre around headache and osteoarthritis – but in clinical practice as opposed to research *per se*, non-painful conditions, particularly anxiety, insomnia, depression, and the 'failure to thrive' syndrome, cannot be excluded from consideration.

The TCM practitioner, faced with a patient having a medication problem – and about 15 per cent of my elderly patients are referred to me for this reason – attempts, above all, to reduce the patient's need for medication. A herbal remedy may be suggested, such as *chitian*, a broth of raw herbs that promotes a sense of relaxation, or the patient may be taught *qigong* exercises for the same reason. The emphasis is on relaxation, because patients are often using too many medications in an explicit attempt to 'relax.' Acupoints that I stimulate to promote a sense of relaxation in elderly patients include H7 (*shenmen*), the source point of the heart meridian, P6 (*neiguan*), the connecting point of the pericardium meridian, BL62 (*shenmai*), a confluent point on the bladder meridian, and GV20 (*baihui*), a symptomatic point on the governor vessel meridian.

From a TCM perspective, pain is viewed as a multidimensional phenomenon pertaining to an excess of pathogenic factors, as in 'burning' pain, or to deficiency of antipathogenic *qi*, as in 'colicky' pain, and the location of the pain is the key indicator of diseased organs and meridians. Headache, perhaps the most common pain complaint in the world, is viewed as a primary condition caused by the 'invasion of pathogenic wind into the upper meridians and collateral' or as a secondary condition caused by 'deficiency of both qi and blood because of irregular food intake, overstrain and stress, poor health with a chronic disease, or congenital deficiency' (Xinnong, 1987, p. 430). This distinction, however, does not constitute a dichotomy, since *yin* and *yang*, the bloodstream and nervous system, and *qi* and the pathogenic factors are in a constant state of interaction. It, in fact, resembles the continuum approach to 'benign recurring headaches' proposed in a recent biomedical discussion (Marcus, 1992).

Headache in my elderly patients is largely a secondary condition, with the tension, temporal, retro-orbital, occiputo, and scalp modalities being the most prevalent. In addressing headache in my elderly patients, I first attempt to determine the disease etiology, and it is sometimes necessary to refer patients with cancer, osteoarthritis of the cervical spine, and other serious problems back to their own or to other physicians and consultants for appropriate treatment. My TCM diagnosis of a particular elderly patient frequently reveals a complex pathophysiological pattern, the elements of which may include an inadequate or irregular diet, the overuse of medications, the presence of a major life stressor, a 'pale' tongue having a thin and white coating, a superficial pulse that is weak and 'thready,' and one or more acupoints that when palpated by the TCM practitioner feel 'sore' to the patient.

In treating tension headache with acupuncture, I stimulate two of the same acupoints used to promote a sense of bodily harmony and relaxation, namely, H7 and GV20. Other points are more appropriate for treating other headache conditions – thus, LU7 (*lieque*), which is a connecting point on the lung meridian, a confluent point on the conception vessel meridian, and one of four dominant points used for treating pain occurring above the waist (LU7 'dominates' the head and neck), as well as EX-HN6 (*erjian*), one of forty-eight 'extraordinary' (supplementary) points, are stimulated to relieve temporal headaches.

I have found this and other therapeutic plans to be at least as efficacious in relieving headache over the medium term (long-term TCM treatment is required to restore and maintain an individual's health) as the efficacy reported, for example, in a recent controlled trial, which found in regard to tension headache that 'true acupuncture was ... superior to sham in only four cases. However, 12 of the estimates are negative, showing that true treatment tended to be superior ... in 12 of 13 cases' (Vincent, 1990, p. 558). Vincent suggests that 'acupuncture could prove to be as powerful a treatment for tension headache as relaxation and biofeedback' (p. 559).

Osteoarthritis, a virtually universal disease and illness in the older elderly, is defined in TCM terms as one of the *bi* syndromes, specifically, heat *bi*. These syndromes involve invasion of pathogenic wind, cold, and damp, and subsequent obstruction of *qi* in the meridians and collateral. The 'wandering,' 'painful,' and 'fixed' *bi* syndromes feature inflammatory, rheumatic pain in the joints, whereas the heat *bi* syndrome features non-inflammatory, degenerative (osteoarthritic) joint pain. The distinction between the rheumatic and degenerative arthritic disease/illness conditions does not imply a dichotomy, since heat *bi* is viewed as a transformation of the other syndromes. This TCM view is compatible with this recent biomedical view: 'There is increasing acceptance that osteoarthritis may represent not one specific disorder but rather a series of disease subsets that lead to similar clinical and pathological alterations' (Moskowitz, 1992, p. 2).

In addressing osteoarthritis in my elderly patients, I again use a combination of biomedical (roentgenological examination in particular) and TCM diagnostic techniques to determine the etiology, pathophysiological pattern, and whether or not a particular patient should be treated by acupuncture. I stimulate a wide variety of acupoints for the wide variety of pain complaints encountered in osteoarthritis patients – to take only one example, in treating osteoarthritic knee pain, I employ a therapeutic plan centring around the following: ST35 (*dubi*), a symptomatic point on the knee; EX-LE5 (*xiyan*), a 'single' pair of symptomatic points in the vicinity of the knee; SP9 (*yinlingquan*), a uniting point on the tibia; BL11 (*dazhu*), a point on the upper back that is 'influential' for all bone tissue in the body; GB34 (*yanglingquan*), a point just below the knee that is 'influential' for all muscle tissue in the body; and one or more *ahshi* points having no fixed locale (these may be 'tender spots' surrounding a joint or myofascial trigger points).

SP9 is a relatively powerful acupoint for osteoarthritic knee pain, because, according to TCM theory, it is the 'uniting' point where *qi* converges on the spleen meridian. The spleen dominates the muscle tissue, transports/transforms nutrients and water throughout the body, and possesses ascending *qi*. In stimulating SP9, the therapist is attempting to 'drain' the excess *qi* so that the spleen may carry out its normal, harmonious physiological functions and patients relieved of their 'excessive' heat *bi* and attendant pain at the knee joint. GB34, it must be noted, is also frequently used in treating sciatica and low back pain (Chen, 1990).

As for the efficacy of these kinds of treatments for osteoarthritis, I have received an 'excellent' or 'good' response from over half the patients treated (see Table 3). These results are consistent with the results reported, for example, by Spoerel and Leung (1974) and Cheng and Pomeranz (1987), who have conducted controlled trials with respect to acupuncture therapy for osteoarthritis and other conditions within the context of pain clinics. The efficacy I have achieved, however, is clinical rather than scientific, and it is assessed by the patients themselves, who are well aware of their own level of pain, and by the therapist, through inquiry, inspection, taking of the pulse, and palpation of acupoints.

Osteoarthritis, of course, cannot be cured by either the biomedical or TCM system, but it can be managed by both systems. Hicks and Gerber (1992), in reviewing osteoarthritis rehabilitation modalities, suggest that the efficacy of acupuncture has not been well established, but Raj (1986b) suggests that it does help relieve joint pain, making the joints – and the patients – more mobile, one of the key objectives of rehabilitation medicine.

The TCM system tends to view excellent, good, and 'fair' chronic pain relief as efficacious, because some progress towards complete rehabilitation is being made, which implies that alleviating pain *per se* is subsidiary to preventing and treating disease/illness (Patel, 1987). The biomedical system, in contrast, tends to view only excellent pain relief as efficacious, a view that may give rise to a sense of failure in the patient, inhibiting her or his progress towards complete rehabilitation (Laborde, 1986). The TCM system relies upon patient self-report and nominal scaling in assessing therapeutic efficacy. This is compatible with qualitative pain-measurement theory, as embodied, for example, in the McGill Pain Questionnaire (Chapman, 1989).

While the efficacy I have achieved with acupuncture regarding osteoarthritis is merely clinical, there are several factors implying a degree of internal and external validity (see Kazdin, 1982, pp. 88–100): the excellent and good responses exceed the 30 to 35 per cent expected biomedical efficacy of placebo in pain relief. These responses encompass a large number of patients having a long history and wide variety of pain complaints who have no reason to exaggerate the relief obtained (the patients have

Table 3. Chronic osteoarthritic pain in elderly patients and acupuncture therapy: Private practice clinical data[a]

Pain (Location)	Patients (n)	Response of Patients (Clinical Efficacy)[b] (%)			
		Excellent	Good	Fair	None
Low back	297	22.5	32.7	28.3	16.5
Cervical spine	253	19.4	38.0	24.1	18.5
Thoracic spine	80	23.7	32.5	21.3	22.5
Hip	74	25.7	37.9	21.5	14.9
Shoulder	71	19.7	36.6	26.8	16.9
Knee	69	15.9	37.7	29.0	17.4
Elbow	64	20.3	40.6	23.4	15.7
Wrist	55	25.4	32.8	25.4	16.4
Ankle	29	17.2	41.4	20.7	20.7

[a] Data from the Steven K.H. Aung Clinic, Edmonton, Alberta, 1986–90
[b] After six to ten acupuncture sessions: excellent = patient reports and therapist observes complete improvement (freedom from pain); good = substantial improvement, but patient requires occasional treatment; fair = some improvement, but patient requires frequent treatment; none = no improvement, and treatment may be continued or a referral made.

acted as their own 'controls'). The data are consistent (see again Table 3, reading down the columns), and these results are in accord with the controlled results reported for acupuncture and other biopsychosocial therapies (see again Malone, Strube, and Scogin, 1988; Patel et al., 1989; Vincent, 1990).

CONCLUDING REMARKS

The notion of geriatric chronic pain has substantial 'construct validity,' and pain clinics should attempt to address this construct in a systematic manner. There is no reason why geriatrics-oriented multidisciplinary pain clinics should not exist, and there is no reason why existing pain clinics should not offer geriatrics-oriented treatment programs. The virtually universal prevalence of chronic, painful rheumatic and degenerative arthritic disease/ illness conditions in the elderly population is the primary, but certainly not the only, indicator of the need for these types of pain clinics and treatment programs. Moreover, it is reasonable to design treatment modalities around disabled, distressed, and adaptive subgroups of elderly chronic pain patients, because actual approximations of these subgroups exist.

The brief description of the TCM system and acupuncture therapy provided in this chapter suggests that both the system and therapy are legiti-

Figure 1. TCM–Biomedical complementarity. From Aung (1992).

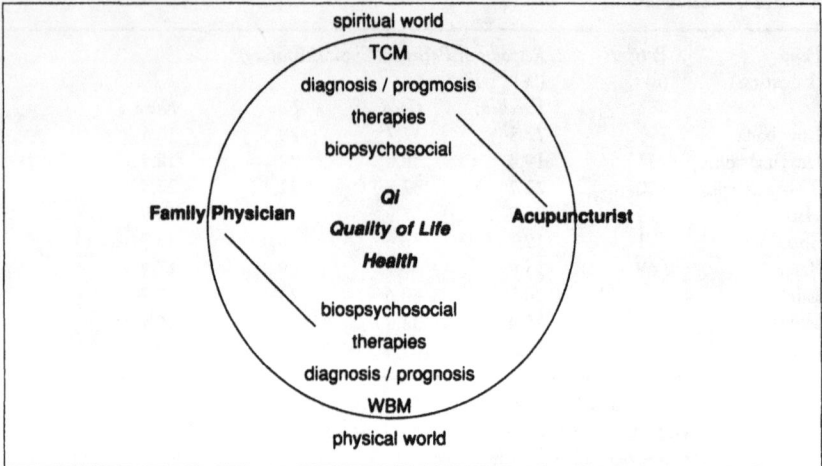

spiritual world

TCM

diagnosis / progmosis

therapies

biopsychosocial

Qi
Quality of Life
Health

Family Physician   Acupuncturist

biospsychosocial

therapies

diagnosis / prognosis

WBM

physical world

mate and, indeed, complement the biomedical system with its numerous, clinically effective medical and biopsychosocial treatments for chronic pain (Figure 1 illustrates this complementarity). The general diagnostic and therapeutic skills of the TCM acupuncturist are analogous to the skills of the biomedical general practitioner, and biomedical – TCM complementarity transcends mere analogy when the TCM acupuncturist is also a biomedical general practitioner who receives numerous referrals from the biomedical system and who refers patients back to that system when acupuncture proves ineffective. Specifically, acupuncture is one of a number of therapeutic modalities (along with physical therapy, TENS, relaxation training, and so on) that should be integrated into a geriatrics-oriented pain treatment program or clinic.

There is an urgent need for comprehensive descriptive and evaluative studies of multidisciplinary and other types of pain clinics that treat elderly disabled, distressed, or adaptive chronic pain patients. Such studies would allow a more substantive working model – or blueprint – of a geriatric pain clinic to be put forward, rather than a 'potential' model (see again Table 2, which is the first approximation of such a blueprint). If geriatrics is to continue as a legitimate and viable biomedical specialty, then geriatrics physicians and consultants should take the lead in initiating relevant pain progams and clinics embodying the biospsychosocial approach.

Finally, it must be mentioned that in January 1993 the University of Alberta became the first such institution in North America to provide a

Certificate Program in Medical Acupuncture. The program features lectures, demonstrations, and workshops designed to make physicians, surgeons, and other biomedical practitioners aware of the complementary role of acupuncture therapy.

REFERENCES

Agren, H. (1976). Patterns of tradition and modernization in contemporary Chinese medicine. In: A. Kleinman, P. Kunstadter, E.R. Alexander, & J.L. Gale (Eds.), *Medicine in Chinese Cultures: Comparative Studies of Health Care in Chinese and Other Societies*. Washington, DC: John E. Fogarty International Centre for Advanced Study in the Health Sciences, 37–59.

Aronoff, G.M. (1988). The challenge of pain management. In: G.M. Aronoff (Ed.), *Pain Centres: A Revolution in Health Care*. New York: Raven Press, 245–51.

Aronoff, G.M. (1991). Chronic pain and the disability epidemic. *Clinical Journal of Pain*, 7, 330–38.

Aronoff, G.M., & McAlary, P.W. (1988). Organization and personnel functions in the pain clinic. In: J. H. Ghia (Ed.), *The Multidisciplinary Pain Center: Organization and Personnel Functions for Pain Management*. Boston: Kluwer Academic 21–43.

Aronoff, G.M., & Wagner, J.M. (1988). The pain center: Development, structure, and dynamics. In: G.M. Aronoff (Ed.), *Pain Centers: A Revolution in Health Care*. New York: Raven Press, 33–54.

Aung, S.K.H. (1992). Traditional Chinese medicine and Western biomedicine – some comparative observations. Paper presented at the annual conference of the Australian Medical Acupuncture Society, Sydney, Australia, 26–27 September 1992.

Bannerman, R.H. (1979). Acupuncture: The Who view. *World Health*, Dec., 24–29.

Bonica, J.J. (1974). Therapeutic acupuncture in the People's Republic of China: Implications for American medicine. *Journal of the American Medical Association*, 228, 1544–51.

Chapman, C.R. (1989). The concept of measurement: Coexisting theoretical perspectives. In: C.R. Chapman & J.D. Loeser (Eds.), *Advances in Pain Research and Therapy, vol. 12: Issues in Pain Management*. New York: Raven Press 1–16.

Chen, A. (1990). Effective acupuncture therapy for sciatica and low back pain: Review of recent studies and prescriptions with recommendations for improved results. *American Journal of Acupuncture*, 18, 305–23.

Cheng, R.S.S., & Pomeranz, B. (1987). Electrotherapy of chronic musculoskeletal pain: Comparison of electroacupuncture and acupuncture-like transcutaneous electrical nerve stimulation. *Clinical Journal of Pain*, 2, 143–9.

Diamond, A.W., & Coniam, S.W. (1991). *The Management of Chronic Pain.*
Oxford: Oxford University Press.

Guillaume, G. (1991). Why Western protocols are unsuitable for assessing the
effects of acupuncture: The need for an evaluation methodology specific to the
investigation of acupuncture. *American Journal of Acupuncture, 19,* 153–6.

Harkins, S.W., Kwentus, J., & Price, D.D. (1984). Pain and the elderly. In:
C. Benedetti, C.R. Chapman, & G. Moricca (Eds.), *Advances in Pain Research
and Therapy, vol. 7: Recent Advances in the Management of Pain.* New York:
Raven Press, 103–21.

Health and Welfare Canada (1989). *Charting Canada's Future: Report of the
Demographic Review.* Ottawa: Minister of Supply and Services.

Hicks, J.E., & Gerber, L.H. (1992). Rehabilitation in the management of patients
with osteoarthritis. In: R.W. Moskowitz, D.S. Howell, V.M. Goldberg, &
H.J. Mankin (Eds.), *Osteoarthritis: Diagnosis and Medical/Surgical Management*
(2nd ed.). Philadelphia: W.B. Saunders, 427–64.

Jamison, R.N., Rock, D.L., & Parris, W.C.V. (1988). Empirically derived symptom checklist 90 subgroups of chronic pain patients: A cluster analysis. *Journal of
Behavioral Medicine, 11,* 147–58.

Jinfeng, C. (1988). Integration of traditional Chinese medicine with Western
medicine – Right or wrong? *Social Science and Medicine, 27,* 521–9.

Jirui, C., & Wang, N. (1988). *Acupuncture Case Histories from China,* Seattle:
Eastland Press.

Kazdin, A.E. (1982). *Single-Case Research Designs: Methods for Clinical and Applied
Settings.* New York: Oxford University Press.

Kepes, E.R. (1981). The pain treatment center. In: L.C. Mark (Ed.), *Pain control:
Practical Aspects of Patient Care.* New York: Masson, 97–106.

Kleinke, C.L. (1987). Patients' preferences for pain treatment modalities in a
multidisciplinary pain clinic. *Rehabilitation Psychology, 32,* 113–20.

Kleinman, A. (1986). *Social Origins of Distress and Disease: Depression, Neurasthenia,
and Pain in Modern China.* New Haven: Yale University Press.

Kotarba, J.A. (1981). Chronic pain center: A study of voluntary client compliance
and entrepreneurship. *American Behavioral Scientist, 24,* 786–800.

Kreitler, S., Kreitler, H., & Carasso, R. (1987). Cognitive orientation as predictor
of pain relief following acupuncture. *Pain, 28,* 323–41.

Laborde, J.M. (1986). Acupuncture treatment: A perspective. *Journal of Pain and
Symptom Management, 1,* 232–4.

Leslie, C. (1980). Medical pluralism in world perspective. *Social Science and
Medicine, 14B,* 191–5.

Loeser, J.D., & Egan, K.J. (1989). History and organization of the University of
Washington multidisciplinary pain centre. In: J.D. Loeser & K.J. Egan (Eds.),

Managing the Chronic Pain Patient: Theory and Practice at the University of Washington Multidisciplinary Pain Center. New York: Raven Press, 3–20.

Long, D.M. (1989). A comprehensive model for the study and therapy of pain: Johns Hopkins pain research and treatment program. In: *Directory of Pain Treatment Centers in the U.S. and Canada*, Phoenix: Oryx Press, ix–xii.

Malone, M.D., Strube, M.J., & Scogin, F.R. (1988). Meta-analysis of non-medical treatments for chronic pain. *Pain, 34*, 231–44.

Mannheimer, J.S., & Lampe, G.N. (1984). Electrode placement sites and their relationship. In: J.S. Mannheimer & G.N. Lampe (Eds.), *Clinical Transcutaneous Electrical Nerve Stimulation*. Philadelphia: F.A. Davis, 249–329.

Marcus, D.A. (1992). Migraine and tension-type headaches: The questionable validity of current classification systems. *Clinical Journal of Pain, 8*, 28–36.

Masi, R. (1988). Multiculturalism, medicine, and health (Part I): Multicultural health care. *Canadian Family Physician, 34*, 2173–7.

Melding, P.S. (1991). Is there such a thing as geriatric pain? *Pain, 46*, 119–21.

Middaugh, S.J., Levin, R.B., Kee, W.G., Barchiesi, F.D., & Roberts, J.M. (1988). Chronic pain: Its treatment in geriatric and younger patients. *Archives of Physical Medicine and Rehabilitation, 69*, 1021–6.

Moskowitz, R.W. (1992). Introduction. In: R.W. Moskowitz, D.S. Howell, V.M. Goldberg, & H.J. Mankin (Eds.), *Osteoarthritis: Diagnosis and Medical/Surgical Management* (2nd ed.). Philadelphia: W.B. Saunders, 1–7.

Moya, F., & Mayne, G.E. (1986). Organization of a pain clinic. In: P.P. Raj (Ed.), *Practical Management of Pain: With Special Emphasis on Physiology of Pain Syndromes and Techniques of Pain Management*, Chicago: Year Book Medical Publishers, 20–7.

National Council Against Health Fraud (1991). Acupuncture: The position paper of the National Council Against Health Fraud. *Clinical Journal of Pain, 7*, 162–6.

Oryx Press (1989). *Directory of Pain Treatment Centers in the U.S. and Canada*. Phoenix: Oryx Press.

Patel, M.S. (1987). Problems in the evaluation of alternative medicine. *Social Science and Medicine, 25*, 669–8.

Patel, M.S., Gutzwiller, F., Paccaud, F., & Marazzi, A. (1989). A meta-analysis of acupuncture for chronic pain. *International Journal of Epidemiology, 18*, 900–6.

Pei, W. (1983). Traditional Chinese medicine. In: R.H. Bannerman, J. Burton, & C. Wen-Chieh (Eds.), *Traditional Medicine and Health Care Coverage: A Reader for Health Administrators and Practitioners*, Geneva: World Health Organization, 68–75.

Porkert, M. (1976). The dilemma of present-day interpretations of Chinese medicine. In: A. Kleinman, P. Kunstadter, E.R. Alexander, & J.L. Gale (Eds.), *Medicine in Chinese Cultures: Comparative Studies of Health Care in Chinese and*

Other Societies. Washington, DC: John E. Fogarty International Center for Advanced Study in the Health Sciences, 61–75.

Portenoy, R.K., & Farkash, A. (1988). Practical management of non-malignant pain in the elderly. *Geriatrics, 43*, 29–47.

Raj, P.P. (1986a). Appendix III: Pain clinics (partial listing). In: P.P. Raj (Ed.), *Practical Management of Pain: With Special Emphasis on Physiology of Pain Syndromes and Techniques of Pain Management*. Chicago: Year Book Medical Publishers, 800–97.

Raj, P.P. (1986b). Acupuncture. In: P.P. Raj (Ed.), *Practical Management of Pain: With Special Emphasis on Physiology of Pain Syndromes and Techniques of Pain Management*. Chicago: Year Book Medical Publishers, 799–820.

Riet, G., Kleijnen, J., & Knipschild, P. (1990). Acupuncture and chronic pain: A criteria-based meta-analysis. *Journal of Clinical Epidemiology, 43*, 1191–9.

Roy, R., Bellissimo, A., & Tunks, E. (1990). The chronic pain patient and the environment. In: E. Tunks, A. Bellissimo, & R. Roy (Eds.), *Chronic Pain: Psychosocial Factors in Rehabilitation* (2nd ed.). Malabar, FL: Robert E. Krieger Publishing, 1–9.

Roy, R., Thomas, M., & Berger, S. (1990). A comparative study of Canadian non-clinical and British pain clinic subjects. *Clinical Journal of Pain, 6*, 276–83.

Spoerel, W.E., & Leung, C.Y. (1974). Acupuncture in a pain clinic. *Canadian Anaesthetists' Society Journal, 21*, 221–9.

Statistics Canada (1984). *The Elderly in Canada*. Ottawa: Minister of Supply and Services.

Stepan, J. (1983). Legal aspects. In: R.H. Bannerman, J. Burton, & C. Wen-Chieh (Eds.), *Traditional Medicine and Health Care Coverage: A Reader for Health Administrators and Practitioners*, Geneva: World Health Organization, 290–313.

Sternbach, R.A. (1986). Pain and 'hassles' in the United States: Findings of the *Nuprin Pain Report. Pain, 27*, 69–80.

Thienhaus, O.J. (1989). Pain in the elderly. In: K.M. Foley & R.M. Payne (Eds.), *Current Therapy of Pain*. Toronto: B.C. Decker, 82–9.

Turk, D.C. (1990) Customizing treatment for chronic pain patients: Who, what, and why. *Clinical Journal of Pain, 6*, 255–70.

Tyler, D.C., Smith, M., Womack, W., & Pomietto, M. (1989). Pain management in infants, children, and adolescents. In: J.D. Loeser & K.J. Egan (Eds.), *Managing the Chronic Pain Patient: Theory and Practice at the University of Washington Multidisciplinary Pain Center*. New York: Raven Press, 161–77.

Vasudevan, S.V. (1988). Management of chronic pain: What we have achieved in the last 25 years. In J.H. Ghia (Ed.), *The Multidisciplinary Pain Center: Organization and Personnel Functions for Pain Management*. Boston: Kluwer Academic 85–118.

Vincent, C.A. (1990). The treatment of tension headache by acupuncture: A controlled single case design with time series analysis. *Journal of Psychosomatic Research*, *35*, 553–61.

Violon, A. (1990). The process involved in becoming a chronic pain patient. In: E. Tunks, A. Bellissimo, & R. Roy (Eds.), *Chronic Pain: Psychosocial Factors in Rehabilitation* (2nd ed.). Malabar, FL: Robert E. Krieger, 21–36.

Vrancken, M.A.V. (1989). Schools of thought on pain. *Social Science and Medicine*, *29*, 435–44.

Walker, J.M., Akinsanya, J.A., Davis, B.D., & Marcer, D. (1990). The nursing management of elderly patients with pain in the community: Study and recommendations. *Journal of Advanced Nursing*, *15*, 1154–61.

World Health Organization. (1991). *A Proposed Standard International Acupuncture Nomenclature: Report of a WHO Scientific Group*. Geneva: World Health Organization.

Xinnong, C. (1987). *Chinese Acupuncture and Moxibustion*. Beijing: Foreign Languages Press.

9

A Comprehensive Approach to Pain Management in the Elderly: A Personal View

GUY VANDENDRIES

This chapter is based on my experience of daily practice in a short-term geriatric hospital in Versailles, France. Over the past fourteen years this institution has treated 2,400 elderly patients whose pain, whether caused by malignancy or not, was but one of the reasons for their hospitalization. The organization of our institution was determined by the need for a comprehensive approach to the treatment of elderly patients by a multidisciplinary health care team. This team is coordinated by a geriatrician. The program includes various medical specialists as well as a full-time psychologist, a full-time social worker, physiotherapists and occupational therapists, a dietitian, nurses, and health care aides, all of whom play a vital role in the management of our patients' care.

In France, relieving pain or at least making it bearable has become a discipline in its own right, complete with a university program. Despite our concern for improving the quality of life of our patients, there remain several barriers to accurate assessment of pain in the elderly. Chronic benign pain in these patients continues to be an area of great challenge for the clinicians.

Awareness of the special problems in accurately assessing pain in the elderly is the vital first step in dealing with chronic benign pain. The complexity of chronic benign pain, particularly given the impossibility of separating its interacting sensory – discrimination, emotional, and cognitive components, is further compounded by the complexity of the geriatric population itself, which must preclude adoption of any rigid procedures. This latter point probably goes a long way in explaining the difficulty of conducting research with this population.

FEW OBSTACLES IN WORKING WITH THIS POPULATION

Two key issues are worthy of consideration. First, elderly people commonly seen by geriatricians are often quite different from those studied by researchers. Usually, the subjects in old-age research are between sixty-five and seventy years old, and they are commonly selected for being free of mental and/or physical disabilities. In this age group many are still independent, and they do not differ significantly from younger adults. Svanborg (1977) in a noteworthy study conducted in Gothenburg, Sweden, found that performances at age seventy were not only adequate on the whole but, in addition, in comparing the performance at age seventy of subjects born in 1903, 1908, and 1913, for certain parameters even an improvement was found in the cohorts born later.

Second, the elderly patient seen by a geriatrician is more likely to be seventy-five years old or more. While the notion of differential ageing is well known, because we indeed see relatively healthy ninety-year-old patients and, conversely, severely disabled sixty-year-old individuals, it must be recognized that advancing age leads to disabilities. An established fact is that 20 per cent of those over the age of eighty have varying degrees of cognitive impairment. Disabilities rather than age, as such, hamper the management of elderly chronic pain sufferers at both the diagnostic and treatment stages.

The following situations illustrate this. First, elderly patients, restricted in movement, are sent to see us only when, for instance, neuropathic pain or post-herpetic neuralgia is unbearable or bothers those with whom they live, who perhaps being exasperated by the patient's incessant complaints want to find out the basis of this pain complaint. Second, taking a medical history even with normal elderly people is often a long process, as many speak slowly, at times going into great detail about seemingly irrelevant points. Some can be very circumstantial in describing their aches and pains. In cases where there are disabilities including deafness or even moderate impairment of higher functions, such as memory loss or comprehension problems, taking a history is at least laborious and sometimes impossible. Third, clinical examinations, particularly when investigating paraesthesia in neuropathies, lose their reliability in cases of even moderate cognitive impairment. We are reluctant to use scales such as the Beck Depression Inventory or the Minnesota Multiple Personality Inventory, especially because there exists a cultural reluctance to take these tests. On the other hand, in the day-to-day medical practice, the visual analogue scale (VAS) is very useful to quantify pain intensity.

Fourth, in cases of multiple concomitant pathologies, it can become difficult to distinguish between acute pain that is new and chronic pain that may have worsened, especially as the intensity of chronic pain varies over time. Here we should reiterate that the recurring acute pain that occurs in repeated compression fractures of osteoporotic vertebrae must be distinguished from chronic pain as such. The phenomenon of multiple disorders explains the difficulty with treatment procedures for the population over seventy-five. Fifth, the quality and even the mere feasibility of further examinations outside the hospital setting depends largely on the degree of the patient's disabilities. In cases where cooperation is a problem because of cognitive or sensory impairment or even as a result of motor or osteoarticular disabilities, a simple lung or bone x-ray can be quite complicated – either by simple problems of transportation to the diagnostic centre or by difficulty in reading x-rays because of extensive kyphosis or other disabilities. Finally, we deal with a great number of other problems in treating patients with disabilities, especially since, disease aside, the side-effects of drugs become increasingly more prevalent with advancing age.

Studies on seniors too often select subjects who are still physiologically young, because they are easier to study. This alters the approach to the elderly chronic pain sufferers and does not adequately focus on the disabilities encountered in the over-seventy-five population, the main consumers of short-term geriatric services.

The second key issue is that many social and emotional factors in the elderly, quite aside from chronic pain, which can aggravate them, can complicate an already very complex picture. First, fear of loneliness is very common, and this is not confined to elderly people still living at home. Nursing homes also harbour a great many lonely people. In the hospital, patients often prefer being in a room with two beds rather than being alone in a private room, even though in our institution there is no difference in price. This is an important factor in treatment, because the mere fact of caring for someone may be enough to bring about improvement. Moreover, it is feared that suspending care can be quickly followed by a relapse. We have also observed a certain degree of jealousy between elderly patients when they have the impression that a doctor is more attentive to one patient than the next. Second, anxiety about becoming dependent (fear of dying is less often expressed in this context) is also common: 'Will I be paralysed?' However, some patients take advantage of their dependency on their intimates with whom they live, usually offering medical reasons for continuation of care. Yet, in most cases elderly persons have no desire to become dependent on their children. Quite the contrary. They very often conceal serious pain for which there is almost invariably underlying organic cause.

Third, seniors often tend to fall prey to a fatalistic attitude. Pessimism about ever getting better, a feeling shared by a number of caregivers who tend to attribute everything to age, is a major barrier in the care of elderly pain sufferers. Fourth, depression, as a reaction to bereavement and social isolation, and associated with feelings of physical and mental deterioration, and so on, is indeed common. Here again, chronic pain exacerbates the situation. The prevalence of depression in old age tends to be underestimated and successful suicides are quite common as was recently pointed out in the National Institute of Health consensus report (1992).

In our establishment all chronic pain sufferers are seen by one of our psychiatrists and, if possible, by our psychologist. Here, we would like to mention the role chronic pain may have in filling an otherwise empty life. One question must always be asked, which can be asked of patients of any age: 'What will you do when your pain is gone?' The contract with our patients does not guarantee complete elimination of pain. Our goal, rather, is to make the pain more bearable. The possible underlying psychiatric disorders are beyond the scope of this chapter.

HOW, THEN, SHOULD WE APPROACH THE ELDERLY CHRONIC PAIN SUFFERER?

The key requirement is time. While this is true for all cases of chronic pain, for reasons noted earlier, it is absolutely imperative with elderly patients. Forty-five minutes for the first visit is the absolute minimum.

It is also critical that patients must always be believed, even if they are not believed or understood by their intimates. Indeed, elderly persons are more sensitive to the empathy shown by doctors and caregivers than to their technical skills. Trust is the essential ingredient of the doctor–patient relationship. Moreover, it should be stressed that there frequently is a discrepancy between reported pain and functional impairment, on the one hand, and the data gathered from subsequent examinations, on the other, owing to the limitations of these procedures.

Having established these prerequisites, we will review the various steps necessary to the good management of these patients. Rigour is vital during history taking, and this is not always easy. Identifying the various characteristics of pain, such as location, rhythm, intensity, and so on, and their impact on everyday life is essential, but the data must be discussed with friends and family members with whom the patient is living as well. In cases where even a moderate change in the cognitive functions is suspected, a Mini-Mental State Examination should be administered during a subsequent visit.

The clinical examination must be thorough, as it will determine which subsequent examinations are necessary. Not much heed should be paid to previously drawn conclusions, except for the purposes of observing the evolution of the patient's state of health.

Cancer, for instance, may not be evident during the first examinations. The slightest clinical doubt calls for further laboratory and/or radiological tests:

Example 1: Pain in the right hypochondrium in a seventy-five-year-old woman was considered for many months to be post-herpetic neuralgia until cancer of the ascending colon was discovered.

Example 2: A seventy-three-year-old patient, thought to be a hysteric because of ill-defined abdominal pains, was discovered three months later to have cancer of the cauda pancreatis.

Neurological examinations must be particularly thorough, as the existence of even insidious focal neurological signs calls for seeking out a specific organic cause of the pain:

Example 1: Parkinson's disease, the onset of which can be quite insidious, can be associated with certain kinds of pain, particularly nocturnal pain, which will respond well to treatment for Parkinson's.

Example 2: Patients with meningiomas (benign tumours that are surgically treatable), especially in the back, often present a long history of lumbago, as the neurological signs of compression remain insidious for a long time.

Example 3: Spinal stenosis can also be found in patients having a long history of lumbago. The onset brings on neurological signs only after exertion.

Example 4: Trigeminal neuralgia with focal neurological signs calls for further probing. Moreover, a neurological examination combined with the data gathered from the history makes it possible to distinguish between neuropathic pain and nociceptive pain, the treatment of which is entirely different. Furthermore, in cases of neuropathic pain, it is necessary to look for anaesthesia or hyperaesthesia, especially when considering transcutaneous nerve stimulation possibility.

An examination of the musculoskeletal system, especially with elderly patients, is of the utmost importance:

Example 1: Finding an atypical pattern of rheumatoid arthritis, polymyalgia rheumatica, or even migrainous cranial neuralgia, can change a patient's life.

Example 2: Palpation of the painful areas, where injections can be of great help, must be done systematically.

Example 3: An assessment of the impact of osteoarticular disease on a patient's mobility and everyday activities will greatly influence the choice of treatment. We should point out in particular an indication of surgery for senile coxitis, gonarthrosis, or even spinal stenosis.

A careful examination of the other organs, followed up with laboratory and/ or x-ray tests if necessary – particularly of the heart, the vascular axes, and renal function – must be undertaken in search of 'silent' illness. Any of these problems can be 'destabilized' by treatment for chronic pain. It is also important to detect any contraindications for antidepressants, such as enlargement of the prostate (found through rectal examination), glaucoma, or orthostatic hypotension, particularly if the patient is being treated for hypertension or has a history of mental confusion when taking certain drugs. etc.

Depression must be systematically investigated. Elderly patients may be reluctant to take pencil-and-paper tests for depression or personality inventories. Moreover, these tests, in our experience, are not always reliable with elderly patients. The long years of experience of our psychiatrist and psychologist, who are integral members of our team, bears out that the best guarantee for accurate assessment and treatment of depression is careful clinical investigation. However, institutions less well staffed could be justified in using tests to detect depression.

Observations of nurses and health care aides must be acknowledged as they have extensive face-to-face contact with the patients and understand their body language better than the physicians do. In cases of mutism, negativism, or posturing, patients can indicate pain through their bodily reactions to routine care. The same is true of mentally confused patients, as this confusion could be an expression of pain in elderly patients. Moreover, the nursing team, along with the health care aides, are often the first to note the lack of effectiveness or the side-effects of treatments prescribed by the doctors. Communication within the hospital team is essential and the doctor, besides assessing the above-mentioned information, must keep the team informed of the possible negative as well as positive effects of the course of treatment.

It is inconceivable that chronic pain sufferers should be approached without first *interviewing their family members and friends.* Their observations about the elderly person's pain is of utmost importance as their attitudes often have a bearing on the well-being of the patient.

SIX PRINCIPLES FOR TREATING CHRONIC PAIN SUFFERERS

Principle 1: set an objective with the patients and the people among whom they live. While it is possible to diminish pain or, in any event, make it more tolerable, one should not eliminate it entirely without carefully assessing the void its disappearance would create.

Principle 2: the organic causes that may have been found must be treated, if need be, with the aid of orthopaedic surgeons, neurosurgeons, and other specialists accustomed to treating elderly persons. The following are a few examples:

1   Administration of corticosteroid injections for a compressed nerve or tendinitis readily associated with degenerative arthropathy
2   Administration of intrathecal injections of corticosteroids in cases of spinal stenosis, or, in cases where the intervals between injections would be too short, a laminectomy could be indicated
3   Adaption of treatment for Parkinson's disease (without neglecting basic physiotherapy)
4   Selective thermocoagulation of the gasserian ganglion in cases of carbamazepine-resistant trigeminal neuralgia
5   Hip- or knee-joint replacement when anti-inflammatory drugs are no longer effective and the patient is bedridden

Principle 3: alternative means of treatment, which can sometimes eliminate the need for drugs, must not be overlooked. One might consider applying heat or cold, particularly in cases of osteoarticular or neuropathic pain. Transcutaneous nerve stimulation is useful as an adjuvant, particularly for neuropathic pain such as post-herpetic neuralgia, in the absence of local or general anaesthetia of hyperaesthesia, or again for cases of lumbago and especially for vertebral arthrosis; unfortunately, it loses its effectiveness over time and, after six months, the analgesic action has almost completely disappeared leaving only a psychotherapeutic effect. Prescribing a lumbar support for rheumatological problems can be of great help in cases of disabling lumbar pain.

Principle 4: drugs that often have already been extensively used before hospitalization must be prescribed with great caution – mild doses at the outset with very gradual increases. The effects must be carefully observed because of side-effects related to drug interaction and the fact that side effects become increasingly common with advancing age. This underscores the importance of considering alternative measures whenever possible. A few examples of problems in handling drugs are described.

Example 1: Pain caused by an excess of nociceptive stimuli. Acetaminophen, because of its few side-effects, is still the drug of choice for moderate pain. However, in cases of painful, crippling osteoarthritis or polymyalgia rheumatica, non-steroidal anti-inflammatory drugs (NSAIDs) provide great relief. Nevertheless, the side-effects of these drugs are particularly common in the elderly and require long-term clinical observation and laboratory tests. Side-effects include renal failure, blood pressure previously controlled by antihypertensive drugs becoming less effective, gastric bleeding, and, more specifically, peptic ulcers (we systematically prescribe gastric protectors or anti-ulcer prostaglandins [misoprostol] in cases where there is a history of ulcers), and masking of infections.

In cases of very severe pain, the rules for the use of morphine-based drugs described by Portenoy (1990) and Boureau (1992) appear to be appropriate. However, the significance of short-term side-effects should be mentioned, especially extreme drowsiness, even confusion, or severe constipation where no treatment is administered to prevent it. We generally use a combination of codeine and acetaminophen, as the two potentiate each other and codeine is not very addictive. This combination is particularly useful in cases where the pain is very debilitating, forcing the patient to be bedridden for long periods of time.

We should mention two particular cases that seem important. In cases involving frequent and painful changing of dressings (for example, ischaemic ulcerations), we use a gas mixture of 50 per cent oxygen and 50 per cent nitrous oxide, or perhaps buprenorphine, a partial agonist of morphine, administered sublingually, which induces only slight drowsiness. It is also used fairly successfully in the acute phase of herpes zoster, but this is beyond the scope of our discussion.

Example 2: Neuropathic pain. The active drugs for this problem have many side-effects, which again call for beginning with mild doses to be increased very gradually. Carbamazepine and clonazepam are of interest in cases of searing or throbbing pain as in trigeminal neuralgia, but they cause extreme drowsiness and require daily reassessments of the treatment. Moreover, the only antidepressants of any value with permanent neuropathic pain are the tricyclic agents. Unfortunately, side-effects of these drugs are very common. The newer antidepressants have many fewer side-effects, but have little or no effect on the actual pain. They can, however, be useful in treating the depression that often accompanies pain.

Example 3: The problem of anxiolytics. Benzodiazepines must be avoided, partly because of the risk of drowsiness, but mostly because of the danger of acquiring physical dependence with extended use. We prefer to prescribe buspirone or hydroxyzine which present no risk for developing physical dependence. In cases of more severe anxiety, chlorpromazine is the drug of choice, because it causes little drowsiness or orthostatic hypotension, unlike methotrimeprozine, which is of interest because of its anodyne properties. In short, preference should be given to methods that do not involve using drugs given the elderly patient's extreme sensitivity to them.

Principle 5: drug-free strategies require the patient's whole-hearted cooperation, which is not always easy to obtain, and experienced caregivers to offer alternative techniques. In our institution, these are the various possibilities: First, physiotherapy stands at the forefront. It is easily accepted by the patients, it helps them rediscover their bodies, it increases their self-confidence through positive feedback, and it gives our physiotherapists the opportunity to teach preventive measures, such as ways to get oneself up after a fall or ways to be careful of one's spinal column while carrying on normal activities. Second, relaxation in situations of high anxiety is very useful. This, too, builds patients' self-confidence by giving them more control over their minds and bodies. Third, we do not use any standard behaviour therapy procedure since, in our opinion, each patient is unique. We do, however, teach patients various behavioural techniques to help them live more comfortably with their pain and deal with their everyday activities. Fourth, for the past two years, with the psychiatrist's approval and if the patient so desires and suffers no cognitive disorders, we teach patients a method of self-hypnosis (Erickson and Rossi, 1979), introduced in France by Godin (1992) and MaLarewicz (1990). Unfortunately, it is impossible to outline the technique within the framework of this chapter. Suffice it to say that there is no ritualized induction, nor any repetition of phrases as with conventional hypnosis. After carefully listening and observing a patient the therapist teaches him, through so-called supportive care and attention techniques, to use the resources of his own subconscious, without the necessity to enter into a state of sleep that can be, in fact, rather dis-ruptive. It is essential that the patient be aware that he is able to dissociate from his body. The results, while still fragmentary, appear to be stable at eighteen months. Meticulous research with a control group is still warranted here, but this has not yet been done. Fifth, the various psychotherapies that could be useful will not be discussed here as they have been dealt with in other chapters, but it would be appropriate to point out that, for a majority of our patients, it is important to find support for long-term patient management outside of the hospital and, if possible, non-medical care.

Principle 6: with this in mind, several complementary strategies have been developed. First, it is vital that people among whom the patient lives be taught which attitudes can exacerbate an elderly person's chronic pain and which can reduce it. Second, in cases of social isolation, we notify the social worker and the volunteer associations who already visit our patients in hospital to intervene in order to create or strengthen the social network for seniors; this is often found wanting, even in nursing homes. Third, we inform our seniors of our availability to them through their personal physicians even after discharge. The discharged patients are encouraged to keep us informed of their progress. Unfortunately, unless they maintain contact with us, we cannot be sure about the long-term benefits of our treatment.

TWO IMPORTANT QUESTIONS

First, are hospitals specialized in the treatment of pain in the elderly necessary? We believe that such hospitals are not truly necessary, as a comprehensive approach is inherent in the care of the elderly patients. All geriatricians must be experienced in treating chronic pain – which is but one challenge of the multidisciplinary health care team. Furthermore, there is the danger that such hospitals may over-emphasize the technical side of treatment of pain for the sake of publishing wonderful research papers on well-selected elderly subjects to justify the institution. However, it could be argued that such an institution would make it possible to train staff in approaching the elderly chronic pain sufferers, for work inside and outside the hospital, which is the next question.

Second, what training should be considered for hospital staff as well as for workers outside the hospital? Along with the university training in gerontology and pain treatment that already exists in France and in a number of other countries, emphasis must be placed on training staff who have long-term contacts with elderly patients, nurses, and health care aides in hospitals, as well as nursing home staff and the whole network of home care workers.

The following key ideas should constitute the framework of the message to be conveyed. Fatalistic attitudes must be eliminated. No disease must ever be attributed to age before reasonably ascertaining that the cause is not curable, whether it be medical, psychological, social, or all three at once. Disabilities must be prevented or, at the very least, compensated for. Risk factors such as high blood pressure or diabetes, which considerably speed up ageing, or sensory problems, particularly hearing or sight impairments, which are great sources of falls and isolation, must be detected, because their existence greatly complicates the approach to elderly patients, whether they suffer from chronic pain or not.

Observations of nurses and health care aides are vital, as their deeper knowledge of elderly persons places them in a better position than the doctors to detect changes before irreversible damage occurs. For instance, difficulty in walking that has not been clearly diagnosed could, if improperly treated, result in the patient's becoming bedridden, with all the problems related to bedsores, infections, incontinence, cutaneous necrosis, and reactive depression. Frequently, such a patient is not able to stay at home, which results in the loss of friends. Chronic pain is but one problem that requires careful diagnosis to ensure proper patient management.

CONCLUSION

It is imperative that we acknowledge some of the pitfalls of managing pain in the elderly. It is needless to state that, first and foremost, it is vital for these patients to have access to health professionals experienced in treating chronic pain. These professionals should have demonstrated skills in detecting disabilities or, even better, preventing them; assessing social isolation, even in nursing homes, with its accompanying depression; and combating the fatalistic attitudes of the elderly as well as of the people among whom they live and especially of health-care professionals. In our opinion these matters are at least as important as access to a specialized technical support centre. Organizations that are highly specialized in managing pain in the elderly are of interest for staff training. Access to these facilities may be restricted, but that does not justify the inadequate care for elderly persons that unfortunately is still common.

REFERENCES

Boureau, F. (1992). Nécessité de réévaluation du risque de dépendance avec les analgésiques morphiniques chez le malade douloureux. *Thérapie, 47*, 513–18.

Erickson, M., & Rossi, E. (1979). *Hypnotherapy*. New York: Irvington Press.

Godin J. (1992). La nouvelle hypnose (new hypnosis), Paris: Albin Michel.

MaLarewicz, J. (1990). *Cours d'hypnose clinique*. Paris: ESF.

National Institute of Health (1992). Diagnosis and depression in late life: NIH consensus panel on depression in late life. *Journal of the American Medical Association, 268*: 1018–24.

Portenoy, R. (1990). Chronic opioid therapy in non-malignant pain. *Journal of Pain Management, 5*, 546–62.

Svanborg, A. (1977). Seventy-year-old people in Gothenberg: A population study in an industrialised Swedish city. (Part II). General presentations of social and medical conditions. *Acta Medica Scandinavica*, suppl. 611.

10

Psychiatric Aspects of Chronic Pain in the Elderly

PAMELA MELDING

> Have mercy on me, O God, have mercy
> Upon me: years and infirmities oppress me,
> terrour and anxiety beset me
> – Samuel Johnson 1777

Samuel Johnson, one of England's finest essayists and social commentators, became increasingly preoccupied with his health and painful illnesses in late life. He became more depressed, anxious, and tormented with his ills, and because of this disposition he has also been described as one of England's finest hypochondriacs (Baur, 1988). If he were living today, he might not have been referred to a pain service, as pain in older people still does not command as much professional interest and concern as it would in younger people. Yet, as Johnson's writing at the outset of this chapter illustrates, elderly people can be dispirited by ageing or illness, and they often have unpleasant psychological responses to both. They may panic at perceived loss of control and develop a need to become dependent on other's compassion and caring. Their cry for help often goes unheeded by the health care professionals.

The late stage of life is a period of major biophysiological, psychological, and socioecological change – all of which can affect the perception and expression of pain. Ageing brings physical illnesses and diseases, of which many are complicated by pain. Some are easily remediable, but others go on to chronicity, because of the nature of the pathology and sometimes because of psychosocial factors.

Given that painful physical illnesses are common (see Chapters 4, 8, and 9) in the elderly, how do they interact with the psychosocial and psychiatric concomitants to influence persistent pain and disability? What do we need to consider when assessing an elderly person with pain? What are the psychopathological links between ageing, age-related disorders, psychiatric disorders, and pain? How do these relate to cognitive, personal, and socio-ecological paradigms to create the total experience of the older person?

RELATIONSHIPS BETWEEN DEPRESSION, PAIN, AND ILLNESS

The most significant psychiatric disorder known to influence the perception of pain in the elderly is depressive illness. Reported community prevalence rates of depressive disorders of 13 to 15 per cent of the over sixty-five age group are considerably higher than in younger adults (Gurland, 1976; Gurland and Cross, 1982), and there is some evidence that the incidence increases with age, particularly for those who are institutionalized – when the prevalence can reach 50 per cent (Blazer, 1982).

The incidence of depression in elderly people who have a concurrent physical disorder is at least 20 to 35 per cent (Moffic and Paykel, 1975). Many authors have examined the evidence linking depression with physical disorders. Berkman and associates (1986) have argued that the associations between physical and mental health are epidemiologically and clinically important, a view shared by Kinzie, Lewinsohn, and Maricle (1986) among others. Lindsay (1990), in the Guy's Age Concern epidemiological study of 890 persons over sixty-five, showed that 70 per cent of depressed subjects reported one or more physical diseases. Depression was especially pronounced if the physical disorder caused restrictions or dependency. A community study of 2,146 non-institutionalized older people concluded that ill health and impairment of activities of daily living were the most important factors contributing to psychological distress in elderly people (Arling, 1987). Aneshensel, Frerichs, and Huba (1984) described a sociomedical model of depression in which the largest single causal effect came from physical illness. Kennedy and associates (1989) also found that the most important characteristic to be associated with depressive illness was a concurrent physical disorder. At follow-up 22.8 per cent of their remission group had improved general health, but only 4.1 per cent with ongoing depression reported any improvement in physical condition. This may be interpreted either as showing that continuing poor health status and persistent disability is predictive of persistent depression, or, alternatively, depression prolongs poor physical health status. If in addition, as is the case with many painful conditions, the disorder challenges body image, causes disability or systemic disturbance, or requires treatment in which there may be untoward side-effects, the person is more likely to have depression (Vervoerdt, 1981; Blazer, 1982; Gurland, Wilder, and Berkman, 1988).

The incidence of depressive symptoms in chronic pain syndromes is even higher. Kramlinger, Swanson, and Maruta (1983) reported an incidence of major depression in adult chronic pain patients of 25 per cent with a further 39 per cent described as 'probably depressed.' Large (1980) reported an incidence of significant depression in his patients of 31 per cent. Both of these studies described a spectrum of depression from major depressive illness to dysphoric reactions associated with chronic pain. Several studies have particularly looked at the association of depression and painful physical disease. Magni (1987) estimated an incidence of 30 to 60 per cent depression associated with chronic painful disorders, and in a subsequent study of joint pain Magni, Caldieron, Rigatti-Luchini, and Merskey (1990) found a significant association with depression. Parmelee, Katz, and Lawton (1991) investigated 598 institutionalized elderly people and found that those who had major depressive illness (DSM-R criteria) reported more intense pain than did people with minor depression who, in turn, reported more pain than did those with no depression. Pain was even more likely to be endorsed in these patients if there was a physical disorder relevant to the particular pain problem.

The associations between depression and pain have been the subject of many speculations, hypotheses, and reviews (Magni, 1987; Pilowsky, 1988; Roy, Thomas, and Matas, 1984; Kramlinger, Swanson, and Maruta, 1983; Von Knorring, 1988), and it is thought that the mechanisms are multifactorial. There is almost certainly a neurochemical effect mediated via the hypothalamic – pituitary – limbic axis which influences the expression of affect and pain. Depression can be regarded as an understandable reaction to the continuing stress of chronic pain. An individual may also be predisposed to deal with stress by psychopathological mechanisms that intensify pain and depression.

Neurobiological relationships between pain and depression in Von Knorring's studies (1988) show that in chronic idiopathic pain syndromes there is lowered brain serotonin turnover, together with low platelet monoamineoxidase (which is positively correlated with serotonin function), hypersecretion of cortisol with blunting of the diurnal variation of plasma cortisol levels, reduced melatonin secretion, and increased endorphin concentrations. Very similar chemical changes occur in depression which is particularly associated with lowered responsiveness to monoamines especially serotonin (Von Knorring, 1988; Asberg, Bertilsson, Martensson, Scalia-Tomba, Thoren, and Traskman-Bendz, 1984).

In addition, there is often a psychological response to continuing pain or chronic debility that is influenced by the interpretation of pain, including the context and the meaning of the pain to the individual. Subjective symp-

Figure 1. Pain and illness in ageing people: A biopsychological model

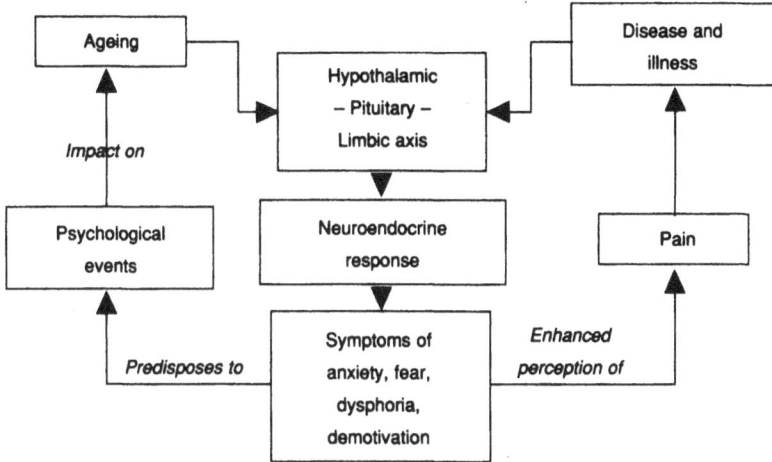

toms may be construed emotionally as fear or dysphoria, cognitively as hopelessness or lowered self-worth, or somatically as due to bodily illness, bowel or cardiac problems, or pain. These constructs may have equal prominence or one may eclipse the others depending on the individual's characteristics. In turn, the psychological events feed back to the limbic–pineal hypothalamic–pituitary axis leading to a vicious circle that enhances the perception of pain and predisposes to increasing disability. Figure 1 represents a model by which the psychosomatic relationships between pain, illness, depression and ageing may possibly be linked through the pituitary–hypothalamic–limbic axis.

The neurobiological symptoms of sleep, appetite disturbance, weight loss, fatigue, and motor retardation are not confined to depressive illness alone, and frequently they occur in many physical diseases and chronic pain with or without accompanying depression. These symptoms are somatic outcomes of neuroendocrine dysfunction, and in the presence of pain or physical illness they cannot be regarded as specific biological indicators for depression. Medication may compound the problem by inducing toxic, metabolic, endocrine, or electrolyte disturbances, for example hyponatraemia or hypoglycaemia, which also can precipitate these same constitutional symptoms (Gurland et al., 1988). However, depression does not just have these physiological components. There are also affective, cognitive, and motivational symptoms. These include the mood disturbance that may be masked by the physical symptoms, loss of interest, inability to feel pleasure (anhedonia), cognitive effects of lowered self-esteem, pessimism about the future, loss of confidence, indecisiveness, social incapacity, and motivational effects of withdrawal and retardation. These cognitive–affective–motivational symptoms are the explicit indicators that characterize depression in the presence of physical illness and chronic pain.

Symptoms of Depression

The symptoms of depression are:

1 Neurobiological: Sleep disturbance, fatigue, diurnal variation of mood, appetite disturbance, weight change
2 Affective: Dysphoria, loss of interest, anhedonia or lack of pleasure in activities
3 Cognitive: Thoughts of self-harm, indecisiveness, lowered self-esteem, worthlessness, and helplessness
4 Motivational: Withdrawal from activities, isolation, psychomotor agitation or retardation

Personal Meaning of Pain

The way in which a person experiences and communicates the distress of pain depends on many developmental, personal, and cultural variables. No matter what age a person is, the meaning of pain to the individual is unique, and it is viewed through the individual's own personal cognitive filter and traditional means of relating to the world. The expression of pain is dependent on these internal personality factors and styles of interaction, which can be considered from different theoretical perspectives and paradigms. These help us to understand why an individual presents symptoms in a specific way, and why similar insults in different people give surprisingly different results. Some may take problems in their stride, while others become chronic invalids.

Developmental Aspects of Pain in the Elderly

Pain and chronic illness in old age must be seen in the context of life-cycle issues. Erikson (1982), Logan (1986), and Antonovsky and Sagy (1990) considered that the last stage of life was one of developmental transition with specific tasks to be confronted. Erikson referred to transition to old age as representing a dichotomy of Integrity versus Despair, Antonovsky as a Reintegration/Disintegration paradigm, and Logan as a reintegration of instrumental (activity, initiative, generativity) and existential (self-concept, autonomy, intimacy) themes.

Stated simply, the older adult has to cope with change in the integrity of the Physical Self and breakdown of health as organ systems become vulnerable to disease and decline. Chronic pain and illness are powerful stressors and invoke strong conflicts in this regard. Older people have to come to terms with their Relational Self with changing family and societal roles, withdrawal from active participation in the world, and retreat or disengagement. Chronic pain may accelerate this process. Decline of the physical body and retreat from the active world allows time to reminisce, to confront the Psychological Self and put into perspective one's experiences of life, its value, meaning, and quality. In this at least there is the capacity for resolution of emotional conflict, integration of earlier achievements, and psychological development – the acquisition of wisdom. The personality characteristics and acquired patterns of functioning obviously affect the individual's psychological capacity and ability to be able to cope successfully with these developmental changes. Failure of the individual to deal with and resolve these stressful conflicts can produce 'pain' in the broader sense of the word leading to the despair side of Erikson's developmental dichotomy.

Cognitive Aspects of Depression and Pain

Turk and Rudy (1986) as well as others have suggested that Beck's (1976) cognitive model is a useful construct for understanding a person's psychological perception of pain. Beck, building on the work of Ellis, originally described the model in relation to depression. His thesis was that depression should be regarded not as an emotional disorder but as a cognitive disorder, in that negative thinking propels the emotional response.

The basis of this is through a series of negative thoughts about the self, the world, and the future that become a darkened lens through which the person views his or her environment. These thoughts create cognitive errors, self-concepts, and distortions that form into belief structures or 'schemas,' most of which have their origin at earlier stages of life. As age advances these life patterns are reinforced with beliefs about the self, life, and health that can become not only distorted, but maladaptive and rigidly maintained. Most of the time these abnormal beliefs do not intrude, but when injury or problems strike the individual, the beliefs resurface and trigger thinking distortions that lead to an emotional and behavioural response. Examples of these thinking distortions are arbitrary inferences, over-generalization, personalization, and catastrophic or dichotomous thinking. These cognitive–evaluative distortions lead to dysphoria and depression, breakdown in communication with others, abnormal illness behaviours, loss of confidence, and difficulty in reaching recuperative potential. Adverse health practices and behaviours such as non-compliance, disuse, and poor nutrition may result – all of which may increase the predisposition to further illness and augment the problem. The model has also been found relevant to understanding anxiety disorders, depressed pain patients (Lebevre, 1981), and chronic pain patients (Turk, 1986).

Psychodynamic Aspects of Chronic Pain

Several authors, including Engel (1959), Blumer and Heilbronn (1981), Merskey and Boyd (1978), and Caarlson (1986), among others, have described quite considerable but anecdotal evidence for the controversial concept of 'pain proneness.' Ford (1977) described a group of patients who fitted the 'pain prone' profiles outlined by these authors. As they developed a treatment-resistant chronic disability syndrome following injury, he used the rather whimsical metaphor of 'Humpty Dumpty syndrome' to illustrate the concept. These patients often had histories of childhood deprivation, premature independence, and responsibility. They also tended to have workaholic and obsessional personalities and often had ambivalent relationships with authority figures.

The Engel/Ford psychodynamic formulation of the pain-prone person is that the person has a rigidly maintained self-concept (ego ideal), and greatly values independence, activity, and caring for others. These conflict with the core needs, which are to be cared for, to depend on others, and to be passive. These core needs are considered infantile and are unconsciously concealed in deference to the wishes of others, and they invoke guilt, which is compensated for by increasing activity. Following significant loss or injury, the core needs reassert themselves, but because they conflict with the idealized self-concept, they have to be legitimized by the implication of a physical disorder that allows the person to maintain his or her view of self and still have core needs met.

Like all psychodynamic hypotheses these formulations are speculative and difficult to prove. Nevertheless, the phenomena described occur frequently in pain patients. Some elderly people seem to be particularly prone to a Humpty Dumpty type of syndrome and I have seen many more elderly persons present with the features defined by Ford following upon illness or injury than I have experienced in younger adults. These elderly people were typically hard working and active throughout life and, when they were faced with significant loss such as injury, pain, bereavement, retirement, or illness, their compensatory defences crumbled, they lost confidence, became increasingly anxious (sometimes with motor restlessness or agitation), felt out of control, were quite unable to relate to treatment programs, and a chronic and sometimes refractory Humpty Dumpty syndrome ensued. Some of the characteristics of these patients include:

- An impoverished early life or strict upbringing
- Long history of anxiety traits
- Physical activity as a coping mechanism
- Previous marked independence
- Workaholic and often high achieving personality
- Obsessional personality traits
- Affective inhibition – denial of the psychological self
- Loss of confidence after illness or injury with marked increase in anxiety
- Motor restlessness or agitation
- Failure to respond to treatment programs

COHORT MODEL

Personality and interpersonal dynamics are shaped by early experiences, expectencies, and social norms, and these are modified throughout the life cycle. As these norms change over time different cohorts or generations will each have disparate cultural influences on their psychological and cognitive set (Elder, 1974). The authors who have described the phenomenon of 'pain proneness' or 'Humpty Dumpty' syndrome are also describing a generation who experienced several anxiety-provoking major life events in their formative years, a major war in their childhood, followed by a world depression, and a further major war in their young adult life – all of which had an impact on their cognitive world-view. Deprivation, both emotional and physical, was often widespread in their youth, and childhood was of necessity curtailed. This generation is now elderly, and these cohort influences on personal characteristics, values, and beliefs are stable and pronounced, and they predispose to certain coping styles – notably those of stoicism or somatization. Many cultures and cohorts of elderly people, particularly in the Western World, disapprove of emotional expression and will present with more socially acceptable physical symptoms, often a pain complaint.

'Illness,' Pain, and Somatoform Disorders

The individual's personal construct of the impact of the disease state can be regarded as the illness state. Disease and illness are not synonymous terms (Eisenberg, 1977; Ford 1986). A *disease* is an objective pathophysiological state or deformation caused by trauma, degeneration, toxins, neoplasia, or infection. It may result in an altered objectifiable pathophysiological state known as an impairment. An *illness* is a personal experience, a subjective state resulting from disequilibrium in states of personal being, social being, and functioning. Disease and illness are not directly proportional to one another. A disease may have minimal impact on a person's state of being, or a person's subjective experience of the ailment may be more than would be predicted by the pathological damage to the body. Disability is the subnormal activity or outcome that results from impairment (Wolcott, 1981).

In somatization disorders, the illness or suffering becomes paramount and out of proportion to the disease or impairment state, and the person becomes increasingly disabled by his or her perception of and belief in a somatic construct of disorder. Somatization is a process by which an individual unconsciously uses the body or bodily symptoms to gain entry into an illness role for a psychological purpose or personal gain (Ford, 1983). There is an emphasis on physical symptoms and a denial or suppression of emotional or mood symptoms. The concepts of the sick role and illness behaviour are fundamental to understanding somatization disorders.

Talcott Parsons (1951) defined society's perception of the sick role as one in which there is absolution from blame for the condition from which the individual cannot get well by will power alone. Therefore the person has to be cared for by others and is released from the normal and usual obligations of society. Expected normal illness behaviour implies that the individual allots appropriate significance to the symptoms, has an obligation to want to get well, and seeks and cooperates with competent technical help. In somatization disorders there is a disproportionate emphasis or de-emphasis on symptoms regarding the objective pathophysiological disease, and the illness behaviour is abnormal. The person is unable to acknowledge the emotional and psychological elements of the illness, and splits the associated affect from the bodily symptoms, which are then emphasized. The abnormal illness behaviour (Pilowsky, 1978) is quite unconscious and of the conversion type, and the person is convinced that there is a physical basis for the condition. The individual thus keeps any psychological conflict out of awareness (primary gain) and also may gain reinforcement from the environment to continue the behaviour (secondary gain).

Use of the psychopathological mechanism of somatization and abnormal illness behaviour ranges from occasional lapses when an individual is under stress to a perpetual, stable pattern sufficient to significantly interfere with normal functioning, at which point somatization becomes characterized as a psychiatric disorder. In the elderly age group, the syndromes of somatoform pain disorder, somatization disorder, hypochondriasis, and hypochondriacal delusional disorder are all diagnostic variants on the somatization theme and are the most likely psychiatric syndromes to be considered in an older patient presenting with pain. However, it should be remembered that in elderly people, complicating physical and mental pathology compromises the validity of the discrete diagnostic criteria as defined by the Diagnostic and Statistical Manual of Psychiatric Disorders (DSM-IIIR, APA, 1986).

Somatoform Pain Disorder

Somatoform pain disorder is quite commonly diagnosed in older people, particularly when objective findings do not meet physician conceptions of organic disease paradigms, and the pain problem is pejoratively labelled as 'psychiatric' or 'hypochondriacal.' DSM III-R was equally guilty of such reductionist tendencies, albeit from a psychological point of view, as it minimized the role of pathophysiological factors in the production of pain. Lack of demonstrable organic pathology does not necessarily mean that the pain must have a psychological etiology. As the work of Wall (1988) has elucidated, regional pain can be caused by non-anatomically correlated lesions in the spinal cord because of the plasticity of the receptor fields of the spinal cord neurons. Use of a somatic coping style does not preclude organic pathology either, as somatization can occur in the presence of disease. DSM-IV has attempted to address these complexities in its new criteria for Pain Disorder. The essential criteria are that pain is the predominant feature of the presentation and is of sufficient severity to warrant clinical attention; the pain must cause significant distress or impairment in social, occupational, or other important areas of functioning; and psychological factors are judged to play a significant role in the onset, severity, exacerbation, or maintenance of the pain.

The new diagnostic criteria have three subtypes that acknowledge the importance of both a general medical condition and psychological factors in the generation of a pain disorder. In the first, the pain disorder must be associated with psychological factors that play the major role in the etiology, severity, or exacerbation of pain. In the second subtype the disorder must be associated with a significant general medical condition and psychological factors, each of which plays a significant role. For the third subtype, the pain disorder is associated with a general medical condition but without significant psychological factors influencing the pain. This latter subtype is not considered to be a psychiatric disorder. These new criteria are also designed to be compatible with the proposed International Association for the Study of Pain taxonomy for categorizing chronic pain. For older people, who have so much complicating medical pathology, DSM-IV's more biopsychophysiological approach does much to dispel the previous dissatisfaction expressed by Merskey (1990) among others with the previous limited diagnostic criteria for somatoform pain disorder.

Somatization Disorder

In a similar manner, elderly people with multiple aches and pains are often labelled as having somatization disorder if physician threshold for diagnosis of obvious disease state or impairment is not reached. However, a true somatization disorder according to DSM-IIIR begins before the of age thirty. It is very uncommon for a classic somatization disorder to begin in late life, as it is a stable life-long pattern of behaviour that significantly interferes with functioning. However, a person who does have a long history of somatization disorder is likely to increase her or his preoccupation with symptoms in later life. Those individuals who use somatization as a coping mechanism in stressful periods of life will show a similar trend, and the early stages of organic cognitive impairment seem to enhance this predisposition (Brown, 1991). Several studies have shown that the normal aged are much more likely to ignore mild chronic symptoms, aches, and pains rather than give them excessive attention – regarding them as the effects of ageing (Leventhal and Prokaska, 1986; Lipowski, 1990). It is the older person who is also depressed who is most likely to express an underlying depressive disturbance by somatization of affect made manifest through the symptom of pain (Magni, 1987; Lipowski, 1990).

The important feature of somatization disorder is the patient's preoccupation with multiple, wide-ranging symptoms. These can include gastrointestinal symptoms, for instance pain and vomiting; cardiopulmonary symptoms, such as palpitations or chest pain; conversion or pseudoneurological symptoms, for example, amnesia or difficulty in swallowing, or abdominal pain; sexual symptoms, such as burning or pain in sexual organs or rectum; and multiple pain symptoms. Usually no demonstrable organic pathology or pathophysiological mechanism is present, and to meet the diagnostic criteria the condition must be severe enough for the person to have sought medical help or to take medication. Despite the denial of emotion the person often appears quite anxious and concerned about the symptoms.

Hypochondriasis

Hypochondriasis is a somatization disorder quite frequent in the middle-aged and older age groups, and it is equally common in males and females. As with somatization the basic pathophysiological mechanism is the conversion of distress into somatic concerns. Whereas in somatization disorders the preoccupation is with multiple symptoms, in hypochondriasis the preoccupation is with the disease or diagnosis. The DSM-IIIR criteria for diagnosis require preoccupation with fear or belief of having a serious disease that is based on the person's interpretation of the physical signs or sensations as evidence of physical illness. The fear or belief of having a disease persists despite medical reassurance. Appropriate physical evaluation does not support the diagnosis of any physical disorder. The disorder must not be of delusional intensity and must have lasted for over six months.

The symptoms often have an obsessive ruminative quality, and premorbid obsessional personality traits or disorders are common in sufferers. The patients are distressingly tormented with anxieties and fears of having a disease, which they are usually convinced already afflicts them. Baur (1988) paraphrasing Shakespeare refers to this as 'Woeful Imaginings.' Emotion is often constricted and cannot be expressed, and, like somatization, hypochondriasis is often associated with major depressive illness. The difference between somatization and hypochondriasis may be very subtle, and mixed disorders exist quite commonly. Anxious hypochondriacs are more likely to present with chest pain and preoccupation with cardiac disease because of their somatic interpretation of the physiological accompaniments of anxiety, dry mouth, choking, and feelings of lightheadedness. Older people are commonly concerned with their bowels, but depressed hypochondriacs become relentlessly preoccupied with bowels and the fear of having a bowel disease. Just as organic pathology or painful injury can precipitate a somatoform response, so can chronic disease trigger hypochondriacal reactions. Bergmann (1971) identified physical illness as a major factor in hypochondriacal neurosis, and there are many examples in history of hypochondriasis arising in late life precipitated by disease or illness. Two of the more famous were the Russian novelist Leo Tolstoy and the essayist Samuel Johnson (Baur, 1988).

Hypochondriacal Delusional Disorder

Hypochondriacal beliefs commonly have the intensity of overvalued ideas, and reassurance of the sufferer may be very difficult, but the belief of having a disease is not usually held with delusional intensity – as it is in hypochondriacal delusional disorder. In approximately 40 per cent of cases there is a previous history of somatization, and the most common psychiatric disorder associated is – again – major depressive illness (Opjordsmoen, 1988). Pain is usually not, but can be, a major preoccupation. The delusion is one way of making sense of otherwise inexplicable phenomena in either themselves or their environment. As with any delusional disorder commencing in late life, it is useful to check out these persons for covert cognitive impairment, as the onset of a delusional disorder may be the start of a dementing process.

SOMATIZATION AS A PSYCHOLOGICAL COPING MECHANISM

There are many reasons why older people may somatize and display abnormal illness behaviours. The psychological processes of somatization and hypochondriasis may enable redirection of conscious focus away from covert emotional conflict engendered by multiple stressors of old age. Focus on bodily symptoms can describe feelings that are poorly understood, particularly when cognition may be failing. Brink, Capri, De Neeve, Janakes, and Oliveira (1979) suggested that somatization in the aged may have the dual functions of safeguarding self-esteem and of manipulating others. A more empathic view might be that abnormal illness behaviour may be the most adaptive way an old person has to get contact, love, and attention, particularly if institutionalized. Dependent elderly people often find it difficult to express their own distress to their adult children or caregivers, not wanting to be 'a bother'; somatization and its accompanying abnormal illness behaviour can serve as a form of communication for some when more direct forms of communication are blocked (Ford, 1986).

Communication is dependent for its expression on cultural and cohort contingencies, and many cultures favour somatic diagnoses and stigmatize psychological symptoms. Old age also brings opportunities for reinforcement of somatic symptoms and society is more tolerant of its elderly being ill, actually expecting them to be frail and infirm. Pain and illness can justify loss of mobility and legitimize dependency (Mackintosh, 1990). For example, it is more acceptable to enter sheltered or nursing home care because of chronic pain or illness than because of loneliness. Political and economic systems also may reinforce somatization by making welfare benefits or accommodation subsidies more attainable to persons with physical diagnoses. Finally, physicians also are subject to these subtle environmental effects and may feel uncomfortable with psychiatric diagnosis and prefer to label symptoms as somatic, thus reinforcing a patient's somatic preoccupation.

Some determinants of degree of disability have little to do with the impairment itself but are dependent on the persons' cognitive beliefs of their ability to cope with stressful events. Coping is the cognitive and behavioural efforts to manage specific external and internal demands appraised as taxing or exceeding the resources of the individual (Folkman and Lazarus, 1988). The nature of coping is multifaceted. Coping can be focused on the problem or on the emotion engendered by the problem. Successful coping depends on a person's sense of control and mastery, whether this is internalized or perceived as external and invested in powerful others or chance. Coping is also dependent upon a person's sense of ability to perform effective actions that will have the desired outcome. Strategies used can be active or problem confronting, for example, active health behaviours, planning problem solving, seeking of social support, or passive, for example, escape avoidance, distancing, denial, reappraisal (Folkman et al., 1987). Ageing brings more and more passive styles of coping (Felton and Revenson 1987; Keefe and Williams, 1990). Some passive strategies such as positive reappraisal, acceptance, and humour when problem focused can be very adaptive; others such as denial, distancing, and avoidance may help explain why some elderly people ignore symptoms or put them down to ageing. Regressive passive styles, such as catastrophizing can be very maladaptive and induce disabling anxiety and loss of confidence. Of course, for many, different styles of coping are used under different circumstances (McCrae, 1982). The tendency of elderly people to use passive coping mechanisms holds potential for development of cognitive–behavioural programs for older persons (see Chapter 4). Prohaska, Leventhal, Leventhal, and Keller (1985) present some evidence for successful use of cognitive coping strategies in elderly persons. Similarly, Middaugh, Levin, Kee, Barchiesi, and Roberts (1988) and Keefe and Williams (1990) have also recently reported successful use of cognitive coping techniques in elderly persons. In their programs, elderly patients who used problem focused, active and mature passive strategies were able to cope better with pain. Those who used more regressive coping styles perceived an increase in pain. Thus, at least some elderly people seem to be just as capable of benefiting from cognitive–behavioural treatment programs as are younger people.

CONSEQUENCES OF PAIN IN THE ELDERLY

Disability

The relationship of neurobiology and nociception with individual dynamic and cognitive perception influences how the pain or illness is expressed and how the person respond to the disorder. The psychiatric and maladaptive psychological responses to chronic pain can make the difference between a a remediable disorder, an impairment, and a serious disability.

Psychiatric complications alter the illness experiences and outcomes. For example, whereas chronic pain causes an impairment, depression can turn impairment into disability by somatization of depressive affect, by inducing neurochemical changes that undermine an individual's resilience (Gurland et al., 1988), and by adverse side-effects of antidepressant or other medications. Depression also may precipitate life events that encourage disability, for example, prematurely going into sheltered care. Personality factors, intrapersonal dynamics, cognitive distortions, cohort effects, and phase of life all may influence behaviours designed to cope with the pain.

Suicide

Chronic pain can be so distressing in old age that suicide may become a realistic option. Seneca in ancient times stated, 'For this reason, but for this alone, life is not evil – that no one is obliged to life ... but if I know that I must suffer without hope or relief, I will depart, not through fear of the pain itself, but because it prevents for all that I would live.' Older people are at greater risk for successfully completing suicide (Shulman, 1978; Blazer, Bachar, and Manton, 1986). A major risk factor is the presence of debilitating illness particularly if it is painful. Catell (1988) investigated successful suicides and found that the elderly suicides had a high incidence of physical illness, and of these the most statistically significant were pre-mortem complaints of pain. Again an association with depression was strongly noted. Hagnell and Rorsman (1978) prospectively investigated 3,000 persons in Sweden for twenty-five years and found that the majority of individuals who committed suicide had first presented with somatic symptoms and pain that masked the mood disorder. Risk factors in addition to chronic pain that increase the likelihood of completing suicide are male sex, European race, social isolation, living alone, concurrent mood disorder, alcohol abuse or dependence, and organic mental disorders.

The psychosocial consequences of pain in the elderly include:

- Depression and anxiety
- Reduced quality of living
- Impairment of function
- Disability
- Increased dependency
- Maladaptive coping
- Suicide

CRITICAL PSYCHIATRIC ISSUES IN THE ASSESSMENT OF
THE ELDERLY PATIENT WITH PAIN

The most important issue in assessment of pain in the elderly person is the need to evaluate any underlying depressive illness. The tendency for somatic symptoms to mask covert depressive illness often leads the patient to be referred to medical physicians rather than psychiatrists. Without a careful review of the total symptom complex the underlying diagnosis is likely to be missed and that has implications for prognosis and quality of living. Unnecessary treatments may be ordered and inappropriate medications prescribed that can compound the problems. Depression can turn an impairment into a major disability, and continuing depression complicating a physical disorder is a poor prognostic sign for resolution of the illness (Kennedy et al., 1989) and a risk factor for suicide (Blazer et al., 1986; Schulman, 1978).

Alternatively, depressive symptoms may mask an undiagnosed physical illness. A major difficulty in assessment is determination of the degree to which the symptoms are attributable to the pathophysiological process itself and how much to a reaction to the pain. As the very nature of pain itself involves both, any apportionment on such grounds is likely to be arbitrary rather than scientific. It is probably better to treat the pathophysiological and psychopathological phenomena as observed. Thus, the neurovegetative symptoms of depression or pain are likely to respond to antidepressants. However, elderly people are often intolerant of the side-effects of tricyclic antidepressants or have concurrent medical conditions that contraindicate their use, and they should be given with care and in low doses (that is, 10 to 50 milligrams of a tricyclic antidepressant) to prevent intolerance or toxicity. The newer generation of serotonin reuptake inhibitor antidepressants, such as Fluoxetine, Sertraline, and Paroxetine, lack some disadvantages of the tricyclics and may prove to be of value for the elderly pain patient.

It is vital to determine the personal factors and coping mechanisms of the elderly person, because these can influence the presentation and perpetuation of a pain problem. Elderly patients with evidence of pain proneness need intensive physical and psychological support if they are to have some return of function and quality of life. This support should focus on elimination of treatable complications, such as depression and anxiety, together with programs designed to facilitate the person's coping and mastery skills. These programs can work as well in older adults as in younger adults, but we should be mindful of the powerful cohort influences in the older generation and that these may bring different life perspectives from our own. Coping skill programs need to be congruent with the values of the elderly person. An insight that a life pattern or belief has been maladaptive can be devastating to some, and it is important for health professionals to validate the previous functioning while encouraging more adaptive coping styles for the current circumstances.

SUMMARY

Old age is potentially a time of enormous physical, social, and personal upheaval – all of which have a great effect on the life of the individual. Painful physical diseases are relatively common in the elderly, and they can cause significant impairment of function. Depressive illness is a common complication of chronic pain and illness, and there are both pathophysiological and psychological mechanisms to link the disorders. Depression, maladaptive coping mechanisms, somatization, hypochondriasis, and unpleasant psychological reactions to pain and disease cause the subjective state of being ill and of having a poor quality of living. Non-recognition or failure to resolve these problems can lead to chronic disability and increasing dependency with worsening quality of live.

Chronic disability, increased dependency, psychological distress, and suicide are negative outcomes of chronic pain syndromes in the elderly. However, depression and psychological distress can often be successfully treated in the elderly giving them an improved chance of dealing successfully with chronic pain. As pain itself is a multidimensional experience, its evaluation and treatment in the elderly deserves a multifaceted, holistic approach.

REFERENCES

Aneshensel C.S., Frerichs, R.R., & Huba G.J. (1984). Depression and physical illness: A multiwave, nonrecursive causal model. *Journal of Health and Social Behaviour*, *25*, 350–71.

Antonovsky A., & Sagy, S. (1990). Confronting developmental tasks in the retirement transition. *Gerontologist*, *30*, 362–8.

Arling, G. (1987). Strain, social support, and distress in old age. *Journal of Gerontology*, *42*, 107–13.

Asberg, M., Bertilsson, L., Martensson, B., Scalia-Tomba, G.P., Thoren, P., & Traskman-Bendz, L. (1984). CSF monoamine metabolites in melancholia. *Acta Psychiatrica Scandanavia*, *69*, 201–19.

Baur, S. (1988). *Hypochondria: Woeful Imaginings*. Berkeley, Los Angeles, London: University of California Press.

Beck, A. (1976). *Cognitive Therapy and the Emotional Disorders*. New York: International Universities Press.

Bergmann, K. (1971). The neuroses of old age. In: D.W.K. Kay & A. Walk (Eds.), *Recent Developments in Psychogeriatrics*. Kent: Headley.

Berkman, C.F., Berkman, C.S., Kasl, S., Freeman, D.H., Leo, L., Ostfeld, A.M., Coroni-Huntley, J. & Brody, J.A. (1986). Depressive symptoms in relation to physical health and functioning in the elderly. *American Journal of Epidemiology*, *124*, 372–88.

Blazer, D. (1982a). *Depression in Late Life*. St Louis: Mosby.

Blazer, D. (1982b). Social support and mortality in an elderly community population. *American Journal of Epidemiology*, *115*, 684–94.

Blazer, D.G., Bachar, J.R., & Manton, K.G. (1986). Suicide in late life: Review and commentary. *Journal of American Geriatrics Society 34*, 519–25.

Blazer D., & Williams, C.D. (1980). Epidemiology of dysphoria and depression in an elderly population. *American Journal of Psychiatry*, *137*, 439–44.

Blumer, D., & Heilbronn, M. (1981). The pain prone disorder. A clinical and psychological profile. *Psychosomatics*, *22*, 395–402.

Brink, T.L., Capri, D.,De Neeve, V., Janakes, C., & Oliveira, C. (1979). Hypochondriasis and paranoia: Similar delusional systems in an institutionalised geriatric population. *Journal of Nervous and Mental Disease*, *167*, 226.

Brown, F.W. (1991). Somatization disorder in progressive dementia. *Psychosomatics*, *32*, 463–5.

Caarlson, A.M. (1986). Personality characteristics of patients with normal controls and depressed patients. *Pain*, 373–82.

Catell, H.R. (1988). Elderly suicide in London: An analysis of coroner's inquests. *International Journal of Geriatric Psychiatry*, *3*, 251–61.

Eisenberg, L. (1977). Disease and illness: Distinctions between professional and popular ideas of sickness. *Cultural Medical Psychiatry*, *1*, 9.

Elder, G.H. (1974). *Children of the Great Depression*. Chicago: University of Chicago Press.

Engel, G. (1959). Psychogenic pain and the pain prone patient. *American Journal of Medicine*, *26*, 819–918.

Erikson, E.H. (1982). *The Life Cycle Completed: A Review*. New York: Norton Press.

Felton, B.J., & Revenson, T.A. (1987). Age differences in coping with chronic illness, *Psychology and Aging*, *2*, 164–70.

Fischer, P., Simanyi M., & Danielczyk, W. (1990). Depression in dementia of the Alzheimer type and in multiinfarct dementia. *American Journal of Psychiatry*, *147*, 1484–7.

Folkman, S., & Lazarus, R. (1980). *Manual for the Ways of Coping Questionnaire*. Palo Alto, Calif.: Consulting Psychologists Press.

Folkman, S., Lazarus, R.S., Pimley, S., & Novacek, J. (1987). Age differences in stress and coping processes. *Psychology and Ageing*, *2*, 171–84.

Ford, C.V. (1977). A type of disability neurosis: The Humpty Dumpty syndrome. *International Journal of Psychiatry in Medicine*, *8*, 285–94.

Ford, C.V. (1983). *The Somatizing Disorders, Illness as a Way of Life*. New York: Elsevier.

Ford, C.V. (1986). The somatizing disorders. *Psychosomatics*, *27*, 327–37.

Gurland, B.J. (1976). The comparative frequency of depression in various age groups. *Journal of Gerontology*, *31*, 283–92.

Gurland, B.J., & Cross, P.S. (1982). Epidemiology of psychopathology in old age. *Psychiatric Clinics of North America*, *5*, 11–26.

Gurland, B.J., Wilder, D.E., & Berkman, C. (1988). Depression and disability in the elderly: Reciprocal relations and changes with age. *International Journal of Geriatric Psychiatry*. *3*, 163–79.

Hagnell, O., & Rorsman, B. (1978). Suicide and endogenous depression with somatic symptoms in the Lunby study. *Neuropsychobiology*, *4*, 180–7.

Harris, L., and Associates (1985). *The Nuprin Pain Report*. New York: Louis Harris and Associates.

Keefe, F.J., & Williams, D.A. (1990). A comparison of coping strategies in chronic pain patients in different age groups. *Journal of Gerontology: Psychological Sciences*, *45*, 161–5.

Kennedy, G.J., Kelman, H.R., Thomas C., Wisniewski, W., Metz, H., & Bijur P.E. (1989). Hierarchy of characteristics associated with depressive symptoms in an urban elderly sample. *American Journal Of Psychiatry*, *146*, 220–5.

Kinzie, J.D., Lewinsohn, P., & Maricle R. (1986). The relationship of depression to medical illness in an older community population. *Comprehensive Psychiatry*, *27*, 241–6.

Kramlinger, K.G., Swanson, D.W., & Maruta, T. (1983). Are patients with chronic pain depressed? *American Journal of Psychiatry, 140*, 747–9.

Large, R. (1980). The psychiatrist and the chronic pain patient: 172 anecdotes. *Pain, 9*, 253–63.

Lebevre, M.F. (1981). Cognitive distortion and cognitive error in depressed psychiatric and low back patients. *Journal of Consulting and Clinical Psychology. 49*, 517–25.

Leventhal, E.A., & Prokaska, TR (1986). Age, symptom interpretation and health behaviour. *Journal of American Gerontological Society 34*, 183–91.

Lindsay, J. (1990). The Guy's Age Concern survey: Physical health and psychiatric disorder in an urban elderly community. *International Journal of Geriatric Psychiatry, 5*, 171–8.

Lipowski, Z.J. (1990). Somatization and depression, *Psychosomatics, 31*, 13–21.

Logan, R.R. (1986). A reconceptualization of Erikson's theory: The repetition of existential and instrumental themes. *Human Development*, 125–36.

Mackintosh, I.B. (1990). Psychological aspects influence the threshold of pain. *Geriatric Medicine, 20*, 37–41.

Magni, G. (1987). On the relationship between chronic pain and depression when there is no organic lesion. *Pain, 31*, 1–21.

Magni, G., Caldieron, C., Rigatti-Luchini, S., & Merskey, H. (1990). Chronic musculo-skeletal pain and depressive symptoms in the general population: An analysis of the 1st National Health and Nutrition Examination Survey data. *Pain, 43*, 299–307.

Marsland , D.W., Wood, M., & Mayo, F. (1976). *Content of Family Practice: A Statewide Study in Virginia with Its Clinical Educational and Research Implications.* New York: Appleton-Century-Crofts.

McCrae, R.R. (1982). Age difference in the use of coping mechanisms. *Journal of Gerontology, 37*, 454–60.

Merskey, H. (1990). Letter. *Canadian Journal of Psychiatry, 35*, 197–8.

Merskey, H., & Boyd, D.B. (1978). Emotional adjustment and chronic pain. *Pain, 5*, 173–8.

Middaugh, S.J., Levin, R.B., Kee, W.G., Barchiesi, F.D., & Roberts, J.M. (1988). *Archives of Physical Medicine and Rehabilitation, 69*, 1021–6.

Moffic, H.S., & Paykel, E.S. (1975). Depression in medical inpatients. *British Journal of Psychiatry, 126*, 346.

Opjordsmoen, S. (1988). Hypochondriacal psychosis: A long term follow-up. *Acta Psychiatrica Scandanavia, 77*, 587–97.

Parmelee, P.A., Katz, I.R., & Lawton, M.P. (1991). The relation of pain to depression among institutionalized aged, *Journal of Gerontology: Psychological Sciences,46*, 15–21.

Parsons, T. (1951). *Social Structure and Dynamic Process: The Case of Modern Medical Practice in the Social System.* New York: Free Press, 428–79.

Pilowsky, I. (1978). A general classification of abnormal illness behaviours. *British Journal of Medical Psychology, 51,* 131–7.

Pilowsky, I., (1988). Affective disorders and pain. In: R. Dubner, G.F. Gebhart, & M.R. Bond (Eds.), *Proceedings of the 5th World Congress on Pain.* Amsterdam: Elsevier, 263–75.

Reichlin, S. (1987). Basic research of hypothalamic–pituitary–adrenal neuroendocrinology: An overview. The physiological function of the stress response. In: U. Halbreich (Ed.), *Hormones and Depression.* New York: Raven.

Roy, R., Thomas, M., & Matas, M. (1984). Chronic pain and depression: A review, *Comprehensive Psychiatry, 25,* 96–105.

Roy, R., & Thomas, M. (1986). A survey of chronic pain in an elderly population. *Canadian Family Physician, 35,* 513–16.

Schulman, K. (1978). Suicide and parasuicide in old age: A review. *Age and Ageing,* 7, 209–10.

Thomas, M.R., & Roy, R. (1988). Age and pain: A comparative study of younger and older elderly. *Journal of Pain Management, 1,* 174–9.

Turk , D.C., & Rudy, T.E. (1986). Assessment of cognitve factors in chronic pain:a worthwhile enterprise? *Journal of Consulting and Clinical Psychology, 54,* 760–8.

Vervoerdt, A. (1981). Psychotherapy for the elderly. In: T. Arie (Ed.), *Health Care for the Elderly.* London: Croom Helm.

Von Knorring, L. (1988). Affect and pain: Neurochemical mediators and therapeutic approaches. In: R. Dubner, G.F. Gebhart, & M.R. Bond (Eds.), *Proceedings of the 5th World Congress on Pain.* Amsterdam, New York and Oxford: Elselvier. 276–85.

Wall, P.D. (1988). Stability and instability of central pain mechanisms. In: R. Dubner, G.F. Gebhart, & M.R. Bond (Eds.), *Proceedings of the 5th World Congress on Pain.* Amsterdam, New York, and Oxford: Elsevier.

Ward, N.G. (1986). Tricyclic antidepressants for chronic low back pain: Mechanisms of action and predictors of response, *Spine, 11,* 661–5.

Wolcott, L.E. (1981). Rehabilitation and the aged. In: W. Reichel (Ed.), *Topics in Aging and Long Term Care.* Baltimore, London: Williams and Wilkins, 87–110.

Zubenko, G.S., & Moossey, J. (1988). Major depression in primary dementia: Clinical and neuropathological correlates. *Archives of Neurology, 45,* 1182–6.

Zubenko, G.S., Moossey, J., & Kopp, U. (1990). Neurochemical correlates of major depression in primary dementia. *Archives of Neurology, 47,* 209–14.

11

Somatic Awareness and Pain Management

DONALD BAKAL, PETER MEIRING,
and ELAINE STOKES

The contributors to this volume have presented strong arguments for recognizing that chronic pain in elderly patients, as with younger patients, represents a complex multidimensional experience that defies single-dimension explanation (Dubner and Wall, 1992). The pain problem often coexists with chronic disease conditions in the form of osteoporosis, osteoarthritis, or rheumatoid arthritis which are all potentially painful (Melding, 1991). Yet there is increasing recognition that such disease conditions, either alone or in combination, cannot account for the widespread differences in reported pain levels by individuals with these diseases. Turk and colleagues (Rudy, Turk, Brena, Stieg, and Brody, 1990) have demonstrated that specific physical findings alone cannot be reliably utilized to account for either the amount of pain or the degree of disability present. Other writers have noted that severity of experienced pain reported with chronic disease often bears little relationship to objective signs of the disease (Afable and Ettinger, 1993).

Because the chronic pain experienced by elderly individuals is generally seen as symptomatic of disease, it is not surprising that they themselves believe that the disease, or some other undiagnosed condition, is responsible for their pain and suffering. Potential undiagnosed disease or injury is frequently a concern, as well as the fear that the pain may become worse, functional abilities decreased, and the necessary help unavailable. Patients also have little or no confidence in their ability to significantly influence their pain levels. The failure of organic signs to adequately explain pain levels is especially disturbing to elderly chronic pain patients, and they often feel that further diagnostic testing and medical treatment may lead to resolution of the pain symptoms. Equally problematic are efforts to treat their pain as manifestations of unconscious depression, family dysfunctions, or faulty thinking styles. Elderly patients in particular resent the inference that their bodily symptoms have no 'real' basis and exist only in their head.

The goal in this chapter is to provide a psychobiological framework for understanding chronic pain in the elderly patient and to encourage the use of somatic awareness as a dimension for integrating multidisciplinary interventions with these individuals. The approach is best suited for the cognitively intact patient who is presenting to clinic primarily for the management of chronic pain. The framework has its origins in behavioural medicine/health psychology (Bakal, 1992) and seeks to avoid the mind–body dualism that can result when mental health and medical professionals deal with the same patient in a multidisciplinary setting.

SEPARATING PSYCHOBIOLOGICAL FROM DISEASE FACTORS

Musculoskeletal diseases are the most prevalent disease conditions affecting the elderly today (Afable and Ettinger, 1993), and some form of musculoskeletal disease is generally present in all chronic pain patients. However, the relationship between musculoskeletal disease and reported pain is far from isomorphic. Osteoarthritis is the most common musculoskeletal disorder, yet only a minority of persons with radiological features of this disease report painful symptoms. Many individuals with significant bone and joint involvement according to radiographs experience no pain, and the converse is also true (Dieppe, Harkness, and Higgs, 1989). Medical experts agree that in most cases treatment should be based on providing relief of symptoms and improved independence. Recommended treatments include physical therapy, psychological support, education, and pain relief through medication.

Providing patients with an understanding of how to manage pain in the presence of chronic disease is difficult. Usually the disease and psychosocial aspects of the patient's pain are viewed separately, making it difficult for the patient to understand what lifestyle changes are necessary to lessen the pain experienced. Devins, Edworthy, Guthrie, and Martin (1992) have outlined an illness behaviour model that illustrates the complex determinants of chronic pain and disability associated with rheumatoid arthritis. Within their model, the autoimmune disease begins with inflammatory changes in the joints which lead to further biochemical changes resulting in damage to the cartilage, bone, ligaments, and tendons surrounding each joint. These anatomical changes are accompanied by reductions in range of motion and decreased strength associated with specific functional deficits (such as the ability to pinch with the fingers). Eventually the development of specific physical limitations leads to more general lifestyle disruptions and interference with activities and interests – a condition termed 'illness intrusiveness.' Illness intrusiveness then results in somatic distress and decreased psychological well-being which worsen the pain present. Illness behaviour concepts are important for isolating differences in coping, but additional concepts are required to explain why one individual with a chronic disease experiences debilitating pain and the next individual does not.

We believe that there are important psychobiological variables that mediate between the chronic pain patient's cognitive/behavioural coping styles and accompanying disease processes. These variables likely involve an envelope of pervasive muscle tension in the region of the painful sites. Although pain-related muscle tension is not readily identifiable with current EMG technology, its hypothesized presence has heuristic value for assisting elderly patients in the discovery of strategies for identifying factors that worsen and lessen their pain. It comes as a surprise to many of these individuals that something 'real,' outside of disease *per se*, might be contributing to their pain. The clinical emphasis on sustained muscle tension, as opposed to musculoskeletal disease, constitutes a significant conceptual shift, because it not only moves the patient away from thinking solely in terms of organic disease processes, but it also allows for a peripheral physiological process which is not entirely central or psychological in origin.

Muscle tension may be at the basis of the diffuse myofascial pain syndrome (International Association for the Study of Pain, 1986). The syndrome is characteristic of many elderly patients with chronic pain and is defined as 'diffuse aching musculoskeletal pain associated with multiple discrete tender points and stiffness.' The pain is widespread, perceived as deep, and usually referred to muscle or bony prominences. There is day-to-day fluctuation in pain intensity as well as shifting from one area to another. Stiffness is perceived and is worse in the mornings. Chronic exhaustion is also a factor and is associated with feeling unrefreshed after rest or sleep. Although some evidence exists for abnormal muscle oxygen tension in myofascial patients, there is no evidence that stress-related sympathetic discharge is the determining factor (Elam, Johansson, and Wallin, 1992).

Rosomoff, Fishbain, Goldberg, Santana, and Rosomoff (1989) conducted physical examinations of pain patients who had neck and back pain of greater than six months' duration and who had poor response to conventional treatments. Patients were excluded if they had received treatment diagnoses of degenerative disease of the spine and/or hips, spinal stenosis, herniated nucleus pulposus, and/or acute radiculopathy, deafferentation pain, and malignancy. They were also excluded if they had evidence of root compression syndrome or positive sciatic stretch. Through this process approximately 50 per cent of the original sample remained. These 'non-disease' patients were examined for the presence of rigid contracted muscles, abnormal gait, presence of tender points, non-dermatomal sensory abnormalities, and decreased range of motion. Tender/trigger points were reported by 98.4 per cent of the sample, followed by 68.6 per cent reporting decreased range of motion, 49.3 per cent reporting non-dermatomal sensory changes, and 21.8 per cent rigid contracted muscles. All of the low back pain patients had at least one category of finding. The majority of these pain patients with physical signs fit the diagnostic category of myofascial pain syndrome.

Tender trigger points are the same as tender muscle motor points, and Rosomoff et al. (1989) believe that activity in the muscle tissue can maintain chronic pain syndromes following nerve root compression, herniated disks, radiculopathy, and even following 'successful' diskectomy surgery. The prolongation of the pain condition reflects, in their words, the failure to resolve the 'associated myofascial abnormalities which produce and maintain the painful state.' It is hypothesized that the muscle tension/tenderness conditions that maintain myofascial symptoms have their origins, at least in part, in the patient's affective and coping styles.

SOMATIZATION

Psychological contributions to the elderly patient's pain and suffering are often approached within the traditional framework of somatization. Somatization is defined as the expression of distress in physical terms. Somatizers, from one viewpoint, are seen as focusing on the bodily manifestations of stress rather than dealing with psychological distress itself. Experienced pain is seen as a way to escape, consciously or unconsciously, from conflict and active coping. The chronic pain patient thesis of Blumer and Heilbronn (1982) is the best illustration of the traditional model of somatization. Pain is viewed as a form of masked depression, resulting from unfulfilled needs. The development of the pain problem constitutes the somatization of the underlying wish to be passive and to be cared for. Elements of this model are evident in the following case.

A seventy-eight-year-old woman presented with pain and accompanying suicidal ideation. Although she believed that she had coped with pain for over fifty years, she felt that she could no longer do so. In the past six months, she had experienced the death of a close friend who shared an adjacent apartment and the illness of a sister who was discovered to have bone cancer; she also had just received a notice from her landlord that she would have to give up her suite after living there for many years. A bout of pneumonia caused her to 'fall apart' with pain and to be hospitalized.

It is not difficult to find the presence of depression symptoms in elderly pain patients. Loneliness, isolation, and loss are quite common. Still, it cannot be assumed that depressive symptoms are responsible for the pain experienced. With this patient, for example, chronic pain had characterized the majority of her adult life.

Current thinking regarding the relationship of depression and pain remains controversial. Estimates of the co-occurrence of depression in chronic pain patients vary widely, with some investigators claiming that few, if any, chronic pain patients are depressed and others claiming that all pain patients are depressed. In a review, Sullivan, Reesor, Mikail, and Fisher (1992) concluded that the literature is more consistent if one examines the relationship between chronic pain and clinically significant depression. Clinically significant depression refers to depressive symptoms of sufficient severity to warrant a diagnosis (for example, major depression, dysthymic disorder, minor depression). Of 623 patients across six studies, 62 per cent had clinically significant depression (range, 32 to 82 per cent). The prevalence estimate for major depression was much lower, but still considerable (21 per cent).

A significant difficulty with these data, as noted by Sullivan et al. (1992), is that chronic pain is associated with a number of symptoms that are similar to those used to make a diagnosis of depression. Sleep disturbance, decreased energy, loss of pleasure and interest, concentration difficulties, and even suicidal ideation can be found in both conditions. However, Sullivan et al. also stated that the failure to treat depression in chronic pain may account for some of the treatment failures in chronic pain patients. Antidepressant medications, when used, are typically administered in analgesic dosages that are significantly lower than the dosages recommended for the effective treatment of depression. In any case, they feel these data are strong enough to challenge the assumption that depression, when observed in chronic pain patients, is secondary to the pain. They believe that it is best at this time to view the two conditions in a state of coexistence and that there is no basis for focusing treatment on pain to the exclusion of depression.

Clinical impressions are that chronic pain patients often present with stronger evidence of co-occurrence of anxiety symptoms than depression symptoms. In many instances their pain disorder is accompanied by feelings of apprehension, increased respiratory rate, irregular pulse, sweating, trembling, muscle tension, and restlessness – symptoms characteristic of generalized anxiety disorder. In other instances, the anxiety is expressed in specific terms such as fear of falling after bone breakage, fear of undetected and/or worsening disease process, and fear of coping with pain without adequate medication.

The incidence of anxiety in elderly chronic pain patient populations needs to be empirically determined. There are community studies that suggest a strong relationship between anxiety disorders and somatic symptoms in general. Simon and VonKorff (1991) used data from the NIMH Epidemiologic Catchment Area Study to examine the relationship between somatization and the report of psychiatric symptoms in a multisite community survey. A structured clinical interview, the Diagnostic Interview Schedule (DIS), was used to assess the presence of DSM-III diagnoses. The DIS somatization scale contains a number of questions that assess for the presence of abdominal pain, arm and leg pain, chest pain, back pain, headaches, joint pain, genital pain, urinary pain, and non-specified pain. When current emotional problems and psychiatric symptoms were combined, nearly 75 per cent of the high somatizing group showed current psychological distress, indicating that one level of symptom reporting is not serving as a substitute for the other. The study found the strongest association between panic anxiety and somatic symptoms rather than between depression and somatic symptoms.

Anxiety symptoms should be carefully assessed in chronic pain patients attending clinics and considered as significant concomitants of the presenting pain problem. There is no evidence to support the notion that anxiety symptoms, when seen in older patients, are more often symptomatic of 'an underlying mental or physical disorder than a primary diagnosis' (Tueth, 1993). It is the case that anxious elderly patients often have difficulty identifying the source of their anxiety, but such difficulty does not mean that their anxiety is organically caused or secondary to depression. Rather the conditions leading to its development and maintenance are usually inseparable from the conditions leading to the development and maintenance of the pain disorder.

Clinicians working with elderly pain patients need to be especially sensitive to the somatic aspects of anxiety. Elderly pain patients often verbalize that they are not anxious and emphasize that they 'have nothing to be anxious about.' At the same time they may manifest symptoms of dizziness, unsteadiness, trembling, difficulty breathing, and chest pain for no apparent reason. These symptoms can operate completely outside the patient's conscious awareness.

A seventy-two-year old patient was admitted to hospital with severe chronic pain that had been treated with phenothiazine. The majority of pain occurred around the perineal region and the mouth and gums. The individual had received a diagnosis of post-traumatic stress disorder during the Second World War and had been receiving anxiolytic medications for over forty years. He had experienced numerous episodes of being angry with the medical system for prescribing phenothiazines. He was admitted to a rehabilitation unit for the purpose of withdrawing him from phenothiazines and benzodiazepines. The patient had one activity for reducing pain and that was to watch television. One evening he was having difficulty sleeping, so he went to the television room to watch late night shows. After an hour he began to sweat and decided to make his way to bed. On the way he lost consciousness and fell to the floor. He insisted, after the syncope episode, that he could recall no reason for the event. Medical review did not determine the etiology of the syncope.

It is a common observation of syncope patients to believe that the episodes are unexplained, even though there is evidence of emotional tension or apprehension within the period prior to an episode. This particular patient was extremely sensitive to perceived staff criticism of his actions, and on this night he was watching television in the same room that the night staff used for their coffee-rest breaks. The awareness that he was preventing the staff from using the room may have generated anxiety, although he never acknowledged that this was the case.

ANALGESIC DEPENDENCE

Analgesic dependence may be the greatest impediment to assisting elderly pain patients with non-pharmacological pain management strategies. Drug dependence has been defined as a 'syndrome in which the use of a drug is given a much higher priority than other behaviors that once had a higher value.' The existence of drug dependence varies along a continuum and the term 'addiction' is usually reserved for severe instances of dependence (Jaffe, 1990). The terms 'physical' and 'psychological dependence' are used to separate physiological from environmental and behavioural influences of dependence. However, in the case of chronic pain, it is more accurate to view drug dependence as an important psychobiological component of the actual pain experience.

Virtually all chronic pain patients have a long history of using some form of codeine preparation. Codeine dependence from non-prescription and prescription analgesics is extremely widespread and yet generally ignored in both the pain and drug dependency literature. Codeine use in the elderly pain patient can lead to a number of symptoms including confusion, sedation, constipation, nausea, vomiting, abdominal pain, urinary retention, and respiratory depression. Even more problematic are the dependent pain behaviours which develop from long-term analgesic use. These behaviours are illustrated in the following medical chart of a sixty-eight-year-old chronic pain in-patient. The patient was being weaned from narcotic medication, and during this particular charting period she was receiving a spasmolytic as a substitute for opioid medication.

0620: Pt reports sleeping poorly, given Buscopan 10 mg for abdominal discomfort
0915: Pt given whirlpool bath to aid in alleviating arthritic discomfort – bath effective in alleviating pain
1000: Pt given Buscopan 10 mg for abdominal discomfort
1100: Serax 15 mg given for agitation
1300: Pt given Buscopan for pain
1330: Pt required much encouragement to go outdoors. She finally agreed, but when she returned she was dizzy and weak – asked for Buscopan
1440: Pt expressing concern about what quality of life will be like without morphine
1630: Buscopan 10 mg
1830: Pt called staff – took a nitro tablet for chest tightness – sitting on toilet holding nitro spray 'just in case'

The same pattern of drug-seeking behaviour and pain complaints continued throughout the entire period of the patient's admission to the in-patient unit. The pattern remained invariant from week to week, in spite of the fact that several different substitute medications for opioids were attempted for pain control.

Pain programs generally recommend making the administration of opioid medication 'time contingent' rather than 'pain-complaint' contingent in order to prevent the pain behaviour from becoming conditioned. This does not solve the problem for the drug-dependent patient and in fact may enhance drug-seeking behaviours as the patient will now watch the clock for the next dosing time and exhibit increased pain, agitation, and anxiety as the drug administration time nears.

Analgesic dependency is best understood in the headache literature where one of the leading causes of chronic daily headache is described as resulting from prolonged and excessive use of analgesic medication (Cantwell-Simmons, Duckro, and Richardson, 1993). The term 'analgesic-induced headache' is used to describe this condition. Although discontinuation of analgesic medication is associated with reduction of headache activity, these improvements usually occur in clinical settings, and the patients are provided with alternative medications. To have the treatment gains maintained in the patient's home environment, it may be necessary to withdraw the patients from all analgesic medications. Most elderly patients are unwilling to consider living without any analgesic medication, as they fear that without the medication their pain will become intolerable. For others, the dependency on medication is a sign that they have real pain and need treatment. Many also have a deep fear of not being able to sleep without analgesic and/or hypnotic medication.

An added difficulty in treating drug dependency is the fact that excessive analgesic use is often accompanied by benzodiazepine use. Because of anxiety symptoms and sleep difficulties, these patients have frequently been prescribed along with the analgesic medication a short half-life benzodiazepine such as lorazepam. Long-term use of benzodiazepines is associated with a withdrawal syndrome characterized by confusion, rebound insomnia, memory impairment, and an exacerbation of both anxiety and pain symptoms (Gudex, 1991).

The significance of cognitive and behavioural determinants of drug dependency in pain patients should not be overlooked, because these patients will often go to great lengths to defend their continued need for 'some form of medication.' Apropos of their thinking processes is Ludwig's statement (1988) that the brain of dependent individuals becomes an organ of rationalization rather than of rationality.'

A seventy-one-year-old patient who had been weaned from both codeine and benzodiazepine abuse during a hospital admission continued to experience 'flare-ups' in her pain months after discharge. She had received considerable training in biofeedback, relaxation, and cognitive therapy. In spite of her gains, she would still waver in her understanding of the psychobiology of her condition, and during a painful episode she would insist that she be given some medication but then would regain some control – only to repeat the cycle week after week. One difficulty was that she was receiving Surmontil at bedtime to help with insomnia – a drug that she needed to sleep. However, the bedtime dependence on Surmontil also affected her pain behaviour during the day. She described her days as waking up feeling not too bad and then becoming progressively worse with pain by evening. She stated that the only thing she could do during the day to ease the pain was to rest, but to rest properly required medication and maybe she would say to herself 'if I took additional Surmontil during the day ...'

There is no simple answer to drug dependency and pain control but failure to deal with the problem severely limits the patient's ability to understand and benefit from alternate treatment strategies.

INTEGRATING SOMATIC AWARENESS

The multitude of presenting medical conditions, the presence of anxiety, and the likelihood of medication dependence makes the treatment of chronic pain in the elderly patient a complex affair. Our approach to intervention is based on a multidisciplinary systemic model with an emphasis on psycho-biological processes that regulate pain and anxiety symptoms. Systemic models are increasingly being used to conceptualize health and illness and are especially useful for conceptualizing the sensory and physiological factors of pain symptoms within the context of ongoing cognitive, personality, and interpersonal factors. Somatic awareness is viewed as the critical system parameter, utilization of which will reduce the presenting somatic symptom.

Defining somatic awareness is not a simple matter. As a concept it is rich in surplus meaning, an advantage in the clinical situation but very difficult for teaching. Somatic awareness has been defined by Cioffi (1991) as the process by which we perceive, interpret, and act on the information from our bodies. To be effective, the awareness needs to be accompanied by an alteration of the sensory symptoms. This state is variously described as letting go, the relaxation response, the quieting response, and passive relaxation.

If one were to characterize the various levels of variables controlling chronic pain in terms of layers or levels, then somatic awareness would constitute the core of the discovery process. Although the concept often does not find its way into treatment plans, it is not a completely novel concept either historically or in non-medical situations. It seems to be best understood in sports psychology where athletes use somatic awareness to enhance performance. Although most human functioning takes place in the absence of body awareness, there are suggestions in the literature that subjects, when directed to bodily sensations associated with their head, heart, respiration, and chest can become quite accurate in the perception of such information (Steptoe and Vogele, 1992).

Patients generally ignore sensations associated with symptom development, for fear that attending to their presence will make the condition worse. They often prefer to manage their condition by staying busy or keeping their mind occupied with other thoughts. In the clinical pain literature, active avoidance through distraction has been encouraged as a coping strategy (Keefe, Salley, and Lefebvre, 1993; Jensen, Turner, Romano, and Karoly, 1991), and to some extent it reflects the patient's belief that nothing can be done about their condition. Many elderly patients view attending to oneself as a sign of personal weakness, preferring instead to ignore the pain as much as possible. However, straight distraction in the absence of somatic changes is generally not effective for coping with clinical pain. Research using cold-pressor task and reaction time attention diversion tasks has shown that distraction alone is not sufficient to reduce experimental pain (Leventhal, 1992). Treatment should be directed towards increasing rather than decreasing the patient's awareness of the musculoskeletal sensations associated with the pain disorder.

Because of active-avoidant coping styles, elderly patients may initially report that attending directly to their body is unpleasant and pain-producing. However, with encouragement and practice, they can be brought to achieve a degree of awareness.

Mrs P. was referred to hospital clinic for behavioural management of chronic pain and anxiety. She had a long-standing history of abdominal and back pain and reported using an average of sixty 222s per week to control her pain and to give her 'the energy to get out of bed.' Medication misuse also included benzodiazepines, barbituates, and other painkillers. She had developed severe kyphoscoliosis secondary to osteoporosis and osteoarthritis. The pain was worse following retirement when she experienced periods of depression and anxiety. Prior to admission to clinic, she had presented at Emergency in a state of confusion, agitation, and with symptoms of chest pain. The attack appeared to have developed in association with her daughter having taken over control of her medications.

Multidisciplinary treatment focused on removing all of her medications. Initially codeine was eliminated and replaced with Tylenol ES. However, the patient's dependency on receiving some form of medication led to an agreed-upon plan to eliminate all analgesic medication. Although her pain levels did not increase, her anxiety levels did. She required several weeks of out-patient therapy to learn to lessen what she experienced as withdrawal symptoms – chest tightness and difficulty breathing whenever away from home. She required considerable out-patient support to maintain these gains, including participation in an out-patient substance abuse program, family therapy, and individual therapy.

Somatic awareness is usually very difficult to initiate into the patient's day-to-day life experiences. Patients will state that they are completely relaxed following the listening of an appropriate relaxation tape, and yet they may have no understanding of how bodily relaxation is to be utilized to reduce pain. Most pain patients do not readily accept, at an experiential level, the therapeutic importance of monitoring their body sensations in the context of ongoing thoughts, feelings, and behaviours. The reasons for avoiding self-awareness are complex and beyond the scope of this chapter, but at an applied level we see the difficulty in the limited success of technique-oriented approaches such as biofeedback and relaxation training when used in isolation. Patients are often amazed at the magnitude of psychobiological change that is required during the twenty-four-hour day to effect therapeutic change.

A headache sufferer admitted to hospital complained of pain that occurred in the form of paroxysmal 'waves.' The pain was associated with a continuous burning sensation, had been diagnosed as migraine, and was being treated with sumatriptan at admission. Since she lived with a demanding jealous spouse, there was a tendency to attribute the headaches to relationship issues. However, the determinants of her headache susceptibility were more complex and reflected a habitual psychophysiological style of reacting towards others as well as the pain itself. While in hospital, for example, she became excessively irritated at the sound of her roommate's oxygen running, felt her head buzzing, and had thoughts of her head exploding. She failed to see the connection between her emotional reaction and the pain onset and coped by either cursing the pain or by trying to ignore its presence. After several weeks as an in-patient, she began to recognize that her head became tight when she was with people in almost any situation. She began to improve her ability to monitor facial muscle tightness both in and outside of interpersonal situations as well as to alter her maladaptive ways of coping with severe pain. At discharge her spasmodic headaches had disappeared, but a low grade continuous headache remained, making it necessary for her to continue monitoring precipitants of facial tension and pain in her home environment.

The enhancement of somatic awareness is not restricted to biofeedback or relaxation training, but remains at the basis of all therapeutic issues addressed during the course of therapy. For example, many elderly patients experience significant pain reduction following relaxing in a jacuzzi bath or pool or applying heat to the painful region. Having patients understand that they are experiencing these gains through relaxation is an important therapeutic objective.

In difficult cases, especially when the patient exhibits excessive use of medical facilities and medication, symptom management may be best attained through admission to an in-patient rehabilitation or psychiatric unit. Otherwise, the patient will continue to seek and receive conflicting explanations and treatments for his or her condition, making it nearly impossible to achieve significant changes through self-regulation strategies alone. Once admitted the patient can be encouraged to participate in a wide variety of interventions including group therapy, psychotherapy, stress management, medication management, and physiotherapy. It is important that one therapist stay focused on the somatic aspects of the symptom and listen to the patient's good and bad experiences during the course of the day (for example, does the pain get better or worse during lunch, at physiotherapy, or during group). In this way the patient comes to understand his/her hospital unit experiences as resembling day-to-day life events. We have seen on several occasions that after several weeks on such units pain patients showed a decrease in complaining of pain and an increased or new openness to a psychobiological explanation of their condition.

What the patient learns through somatic awareness interventions is not necessarily known. Unlike the athlete who is learning a specific skill for a particular application, the patient needs to use this awareness in all aspects of waking and sleeping life. In some instances, patients simply cannot develop the concept within themselves to a significant degree. The elderly syncope patient cited earlier could not easily identify somatic cues that marked the onset of syncope. As an in-patient he was intellectually fascinated with passive relaxation and with EMG biofeedback, yet during training sessions there was no experiential awareness of changing EMG levels. At the beginning of the session, he could raise the levels higher only by making a fist followed by opening his fist and watching the EMG metre levels fall. He could not experience these changes beyond watching the values rise and fall on the metre. He also found it impossible to breathe diaphragmatically. The patient attributed his difficulties to the lifelong use of medication. During the course of therapy he was able to identify external situations in which he was 'uptight,' and he became better, in his words, at 'walking away' from these situations.

We have outlined a systemic psychobiological approach to therapy which places somatic awareness at the core. The concept provides therapists with an understanding that incorporates physiological, cognitive, behavioural, and interactional processes. The key to symptom management remains becoming more rather than less aware of body sensations that accompany thoughts, feelings, and behaviours. Somatization patients have an especially difficult time grasping the distinction between preoccupation with their symptom and appropriate somatic awareness. Unresolved medical concerns, fears of functioning without medication, personality and self-esteem issues, and interpersonal problems all add to the difficulty but can still be addressed with the goal of increasing awareness in mind. The more complex the patient, the more multidimensional the interventions need to be.

The heuristic value of somatic awareness lies in its ability to integrate a number of determinants of somatic symptoms within a single framework. In seeking medical intervention, these patients often believe that they have no role to play in the alleviation of their symptoms. Efforts to explain their symptom as being caused by depression often fare no better, as the patients resent the implication that they have a psychological problem. They must come to understand that their symptoms have a physiological substrate and that the symptoms are inextricably tied to their thoughts, feelings, and bodily sensations. Regulating the complex processes involved is best guided by developing enduring and over-riding habits of somatic awareness.

REFERENCES

Afable, R.F., & Ettinger, W.H. (1993). Musculoskeletal disease in the aged: Diagnosis and management. *Drugs and Aging, 3*, 49–59.

Bakal, D.A. (1992). *Psychology and health* (2nd ed.). New York: Springer.

Blumer. D., & Heilbronn, M. (1982). Chronic pain as a variant of depressive disease: The pain-prone disorder. *Journal of Nervous and Mental Disease, 170*, 381–406.

Cantwell-Simmons, E., Duckro, P.N., & Richardson, W.D. (1993). A review of studies on the relationships of chronic analgesic use and chronic headaches. *Headache Quarterly: Current Treatment and Research, 4*, 28–35.

Cioffi, D. (1991). Beyond attentional strategies: A cognitive–perceptual model of somatic interpretation. *Psychological Bulletin, 109*, 25–41.

Devins, G.M., Edworthy, S.M., Guthrie, N.G. & Martin, L. (1992). Illness intrusiveness in rheumatoid arthritis: Differential impact on depressive symptoms over the adult lifespan. *Journal of Rheumatology, 19*, 709–15.

Dieppe, P.A., Harkness, J.A.L., & Higgs, E.R. (1989). Osteoarthritis. In:

P.D. Wall, & R. Melzack (Eds.), *Textbook of Pain* (2nd ed.). London: Churchill Livingstone, 306–16.

Dubner,R., & Wall, P.D. (1992). Editorial comment. *Pain, 50,* 1.

Elam, M., Johansson, G., & Wallin, B.G. (1992). Do patients with primary fibromyalgia have an altered muscle sympathetic nerve activity? *Pain, 48,* 371–5.

Gudex, C. (1991). Adverse effects of benzodiazepines. *Social Science and Medicine, 33,* 587–96.

International Association for the Study of Pain (1986). *Classification of Chronic Pain.* Seattle: IASP Publications.

Jaffe, J.H. (1990). Drug addiction and drug abuse. In: A.G. Gilman, T.W. Rell, A.S. Nos, & P. Taylor (Eds.), *Goodman and Gilman's The Pharmacological Basis of Therepeutics (8th ed.).* New York: Pergamon Press, 522–73.

Jensen, M.P., Turner, J.A., Romano, J.M., & Karoly, P. (1991). Coping with chronic pain: A critical review of the literature. *Pain, 47,* 249–83.

Keefe, F.J., Salley, Jr, A.N., & Lefebvre, J.C. (1993). Coping with pain: Conceptual concerns and future directions. *Pain, 51,* 131–4,

Leventhal, H. (1992). I know distraction works even though it doesn't! *Health Psychology, 11,* 208–9.

Ludwig, A.M. (1988). *Understanding the Alcoholic's Mind: The Nature of Craving and How to Control It.* New York: Oxford University Press.

Melding, P.S. (1991). Is there such a thing as geriatric pain? *Pain, 46,* 119–21.

Rosomoff, H.L., Fishbain, D.A., Goldberg, M., Santana, R., & Rosomoff, R.S. (1989). Physical findings in patients with chronic intractable benign pain of the neck and/or back. *Pain, 37,* 279–87.

Rudy, T.E., Turk, D.C., Brena, S.F., Stieg, R.L., & Brody, M.C. (1990). Quantification of biomedical findings of chronic pain patients: Development of an index of pathology. *Pain, 42,* 167–82.

Simon, G.E., & VonKorff, M. (1991). Somatization and psychiatric disorder in the NIMH Epidemiologic Catchment Area Study. *American Journal of Psychiatry, 148,* 1494–500.

Steptoe, A., & Vogele, C. (1992). Individual differences in the perception of bodily sensations: The role of trait anxiety and coping style. *Behaviour Research and Therapy, 30,* 597–607.

Sullivan, M.J.L., Reesor, K., Mikail, S., & Fisher, R. (1992). The treatment of depression in chronic low back pain: Review and recommendations. *Pain, 50,* 5–13.

Tueth, M.J. (1993). Anxiety in the older patient: Differential diagnosis and treatment. *Geriatrics, 48,* 51–4.

www.ingramcontent.com/pod-product-compliance
Lightning Source LLC
Chambersburg PA
CBHW020833210326
41598CB00019B/1883